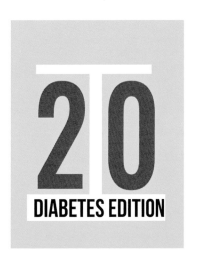

DR. FUHRMAN'S TRANSFORMATION 20 DIABETES
REDUCE OR ELIMINATE TYPE 2 DIABETES AND LOSE WEIGHT IN 20 DAYS

Joel Fuhrman, M.D.

Published by:
Gift of Health Press

FOREWORD

I am proud to offer you the opportunity to enjoy better health and to feel more energetic than you have in years. A diagnosis of type 2 diabetes can be devastating. However, in most cases, this disease can be completely reversed — and prevented from recurring – through dietary intervention. By eating a nutrient-dense, plant-rich diet, you can achieve sustainable weight loss, enabling dramatic improvements to your health.

My approach has been proven to work. I will show you how your body can heal itself when it has the necessary nutrients. I have seen this happen over and over in my 25-plus years practicing nutritional medicine. This program offers you freedom from medication, adds years to your life and gives you the energy you thought was gone forever. Following through on the strategies I propose here can be the best decision you will ever make for yourself, and

should spur you on to continue to eat healthfully and avoid the complications that often loom for individuals with type 2 diabetes.

Most importantly, this program must be started under medical supervision. If you are currently on type 2 diabetes medication, it is crucial to consult with your physician before you embark on this plan. You and your physician have to outline how to gradually lower your medication, so you do not become dangerously overmedicated. This program will lower your blood glucose and blood pressure dramatically. It is vital that you consult with your physician during this process, since, as your blood glucose and blood pressure begin to reach healthier levels, it can place you at risk if you don't change the dose of medication you are on. In most cases, with long-term adherence to this program, all medications can eventually be discontinued as you

lose weight and improve your health.

This program is best utilized in conjunction with the information you will learn in my book *The End of Diabetes*. It takes the right information to beat diabetes and heart disease for good.

A health transformation is yours to attain in 20 days. I hope your results will encourage and motivate you to continue to eat healthfully for the rest of your life.

Wishing you the best of health always,

Joel Fuhrman

TABLE OF CONTENTS

Introduction 1

Connections..3

Why the Nutritarian Diet Works............................4

The Best and Worst Foods For Diabetics 5

The Importance of Glycemic Load 7

Frequently Asked Questions................................8

Important Supplements......................................11

Get Moving 13

The Ground Rules...14

Foods to Eat Liberally, Eat in Moderation,
or Avoid Entirely..15

Stock Your Pantry 16

Shopping List (Days 1 to 5)...............................17

Meal Plan and Recipes (Days 1 to 5).................18

Shopping List (Days 6 to 10)..............................25

Meal Plan and Recipes (Days 6 to 10)................26

Shopping List (Days 11 to 15) 35

Meal Plan and Recipes (Days 11 to 15)..............36

Shopping List (Days 16 to 20) 41

Meal Plan and Recipes (Days 16 to 20)..............42

Congratulations! 49

What's Next?..50

Dr. Fuhrman's Additional Services.....................51

Eat to Live Retreat 52

References..53

About Joel Fuhrman, M.D..................................55

INTRODUCTION

LET'S FACE IT:

TYPE 2 DIABETES CAN BE AN OVERWHELMING DISEASE.

You probably searched the internet for information when you were diagnosed. No doubt some of it was scary. But now your focus should be on learning how type 2 diabetes can be improved – and in most cases, reversed – so you are no longer diabetic, through Nutritarian dietary intervention. This transformation, from the throes of the disease to wellness, can be quick, and it can be permanent.

That's right. It is possible (with your doctor's guidance) to gradually reduce and eventually free yourself from the medications, glucose monitoring, HbA1C measurements, medical appointments, and devastating complications tied to this life-threatening disease. All of this is possible if you are committed to addressing the underlying cause of the disease – your diet. To put it simply: Food got you into this mess, and food can surely get you out.

Transformation 20 Diabetes Edition is a targeted program that allows most people to reduce or eliminate their diabetes medication in 20 days. This program is designed for people who want to take aggressive action in their battle against type 2 diabetes. By strictly following the meal plans, you will lose weight, reverse your diabetes and lower your blood pressure. You will also begin to reduce your risk of cardiovascular disease, boost your immunity to common illnesses and increase your longevity.

WHY MEDICATION ISN'T ENOUGH

Commitment is key. When the going gets a little tough, I need you to hang in there. Here's why: Managing diabetes with medication is just that; you are *managing* it. There is no chance of reversing it, and the possibility of eventual complications associated with diabetes remains the same. Nutritional management of the disease – even if you are only able to reduce your medication and not eliminate it – is the only way you will be able to reduce your risk of cardiovascular disease and other complications. Medication alone will not provide the same protection. Medication keeps blood glucose under control, but it can't restore your health the way healthy living can. Losing weight, flooding your body with the micronutrients it has been missing, and lowering inflammation are all key to your future health.

Following my program is a commitment to take control of your health and lifestyle. In less than three weeks you can be on the road back to better health. Think about that. Instead of disease control, your goal can be disease reversal, potentially eliminating the disease from your life forever.

NUTRITION IS THE PRESCRIPTION

A nutritional approach to type 2 diabetes has been proven to stabilize blood sugar and reduce or eliminate the need for medication. In a study of patients with type 2 diabetes, 90 percent of those following a high-nutrient, low-glycemic diet were able to eliminate all of their medications for diabetes, and their mean HbA1c after one year was 5.8 percent, which is within the normal range.[1] A high-nutrient, low-glycemic diet is one that is rich in vegetables, nuts, seeds, beans, and some fresh fruits, and that limits meat and grains. This type of diet has been proven to not only prevent and reverse disease, but foster long-term health.

In my book *The End of Diabetes*, I discuss in detail how superior nutrition can reverse type 2 diabetes, and how those with type 1 diabetes can improve their health and quality of life through a high-nutrient, plant-rich diet. Transformation 20 is a quick start on the road to excellent, sustainable health. But it doesn't end here. I urge you to really explore what it means to be healthy and how to eat for long-term wellness, by reading *The End of Diabetes*. It will allow you to more fully understand why a Nutritarian diet works so well.

Make *Transformation 20* the beginning of a whole new lifestyle. Invest in yourself. You won't be sorry.

I get it. Changing your diet after decades of eating a certain way may seem difficult. But this really can be an issue of life or death. The key is to adapt a diet that can be healthful and — this is crucial — sustainable. I have designed *Transformation 20 Diabetes* to suppress your appetite and reduce food cravings. Strictly following this program will allow you to reset your palate and allow you to savor the flavors of natural food.

WHAT'S THE CATCH?

There isn't one. The nutritional plan that I outline in this book is one that I have used successfully with thousands of my patients for more than 25 years. It is designed to address the specific and urgent health challenges of type 2 diabetics and to resolve them quickly. My approach has been proven to work. You will swiftly see radical improvement to your health while achieving safe weight loss. All you need is the commitment to see it through. You have taken the first step — which is often the hardest. Let's begin the rest of the process now.

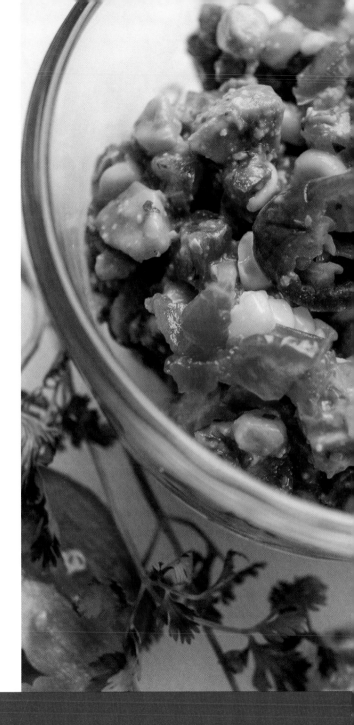

CONNECTIONS

You aren't alone on this journey! An important part of the *Transformation 20* program is your ability to connect with those going through the same process. Use this support to lean on others to keep you going and accountable. Get advice and compare notes, and you won't be derailed.

By purchasing this program you'll also be able to join the private Dr. Fuhrman T20 Diabetes Facebook page, where you can interact with others following the *Transformation 20 Diabetes* program. It is a great place to share tips, trade recipes and get inspired! Join now: www.facebook.com/groups/DrFuhrmanT20Diabetes

In addition, membership to DrFuhrman.com will give you access to a wealth of health and nutrition resources, including a Health Tracker so you can monitor your progress, the Nutritarian Recipe Database with more than 1,700 recipes, and a dedicated Transformation 20 Diabetes Community where you can post questions. You will also have access to our Ask the Doctor forum, plus other exclusive perks. www.DrFuhrman.com/membership.

SHOPPING TIP

The ingredients for all of the recipes in this plan are available at your favorite food markets. But it can be a challenge to find prepared foods, such as salad dressings, soups and condiments, that are made without added salt, sugar, oils and starches. You'll find these products, as well as multivitamins, supplements, books and media in our shop at **DrFuhrman.com**.

TESTIMONIAL

At 6'1" Scott was 270 pounds and was diagnosed with type 2 diabetes. He had blood pressure of 201/110, a blood glucose level of 385 with an HbA1C level of 11, and a cholesterol reading of 270. To put it mildly, Scott was very ill. His doctor prescribed five different medicines. Desperate to help him, his wife started researching what Scott should eat and she came across information on Dr. Fuhrman's Nutritarian diet. Instead of five medicines to control his diabetes, Scott used the Nutritarian diet to reverse his diabetes.

Scott not only lost 60 pounds, but his high blood pressure and diabetes are gone. Look at his new numbers–blood pressure is now 107/78, blood glucose of 83, HbA1C level of 5, and total cholesterol of 130.

"Dr. Fuhrman's help has led me to a healthy lifestyle that is so wonderful for me and my wife," Scott says. "Thanks, Dr. Fuhrman!"

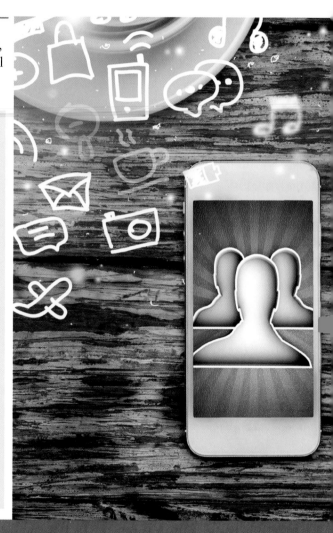

WHY THE NUTRITARIAN DIET WORKS FOR TYPE 2 DIABETICS

Treating type 2 diabetes with medication without changing your diet is a failed approach. The majority of medications used to lower blood sugar place stress on your already-failing pancreas. In addition, these medications have serious side effects. Some increase the risk of kidney dysfunction, heart failure, and cancer. Some also cause weight gain, and over time, worsen diabetes. It's a vicious cycle. As you gain weight, you become more insulin resistant, and you need more medication. Your pancreas pushes to meet these higher insulin demands and eventually can't. After that, you may need to take insulin, too.

I developed the Nutritarian eating style to harness the body's tremendous power to heal itself through proper nutrition. Many conventional diabetes diets rely on meat and other animal products as the major source of calories to keep glycemic effects down. This strategy has serious drawbacks. Those diets actually promote inflammation and oxidative stress and lead to weight gain, diabetes and heart disease.[2-6] High animal-protein diets are linked to cancer and premature death.[7, 8] Only a Nutritarian diet can facilitate the dramatic – and permanent – weight loss your body needs to repair damaged cells caused by type 2 diabetes and significantly improve your quality of life, giving you more energy and vitality. At the same time, a Nutritarian diet lowers your risk of cancer.

This program is nutrient dense and plant rich, utilizing lots of whole plant foods like vegetables, mushrooms, beans, nuts, seeds and some fruit. These foods supply essential macronutrients (protein, carbohydrates and fat) and vital micronutrients (vitamins, phytochemicals and minerals).

This way of eating maximizes your body's natural ability to self-heal and repair. You will be eliminating foods that are completely empty of nutrients, such as sugar, sweeteners, white flour and processed foods.

My recommendations call for eating larger quantities of nutrient-rich foods and fewer foods with low nutritional value. You will see that as you begin this way of eating and your body responds to getting proper nutrition, your appetite for empty-calorie foods will decrease, your desire to overeat will be curtailed, and your craving for junk foods will lessen.

If you have tried other diets and failed, don't despair. This program lessens and resolves food addictions and emotional overeating. It has worked time and again for those in your shoes. And, don't assume that good health and an ideal weight are the result of genetics or luck. The reality is that we bear responsibility for our own health and appearance through the dietary choices we make. Strictly following these meal plans makes it easy to realize success quickly, introduces you to some of the principles of the Nutritarian eating style, and helps you to understand that this is not a one-time diet. It is a lifestyle – one that you can successfully embrace.

NUTRITARIAN BENEFITS:
- REDUCE OR ELIMINATE TYPE 2 DIABETES MEDICATIONS IN 20 DAYS
- RESTORE INSULIN SENSITIVITY
- LOWER BLOOD GLUCOSE NUMBERS
- IMPROVE PANCREATIC FUNCTION
- LOSE WEIGHT – OFTEN MORE THAN 10 POUNDS IN 20 DAYS
- LOWER BLOOD PRESSURE AND CHOLESTEROL
- REVERSE ATHEROSCLEROSIS (BLOOD VESSEL PLAQUE)
- ESTABLISH NEW EATING HABITS AND TASTE PREFERENCES
- REGAIN ENERGY
- PROTECT AGAINST HEART DISEASE, STROKE AND OTHER SERIOUS ILLNESSES

THE BEST & WORST
FOODS FOR DIABETICS

Your food choices can either prevent or promote insulin resistance and type 2 diabetes. As adults, we often like the foods we were raised with best. But continuing to eat only the foods you are familiar with can be your downfall.

My advice for your success is: **Be a choosy eater, not a picky one.** Research shows that it takes between eight to fifteen times of eating a new food to accept it as familiar. Taste is a learned pattern. Repeated exposure to a variety of fruits and vegetables has been shown to increase our acceptance and liking of them. So, if you find a food on the 'Best' list that has you turning up your nose, give it another try and keep trying.

For now, I would like you to accept the notion that I will choose what you will eat, not you. It makes it easy, because the decision is made for you, and the results will amaze you. Over time, you will like these foods more and more. Just keep on doing it, and soon you will be lovin' it.

THE BEST FOODS

High-nutrient, low-glycemic-load (GL) foods are optimal for people with diabetes, and these foods also help to prevent type 2 diabetes from developing in the first place.

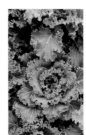

GREEN VEGETABLES

Leafy greens, cruciferous and other green vegetables are the most important foods to focus on for diabetes reversal and prevention. Higher green vegetable consumption is associated with lower HbA1c levels.[9]

NON-GREEN, NON-STARCHY VEGETABLES

Mushrooms, onions, garlic, eggplant, peppers, tomatoes, cauliflower, and other non-green, non-starchy vegetables have almost no effect on blood glucose.

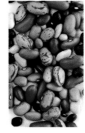

BEANS, LENTILS, AND OTHER LEGUMES

Due to their moderate protein and high fiber and resistant starch content, beans are the ideal carbohydrate and have a low glycemic load. They are also an ideal weight-loss food, as our digestive system is unable to absorb all the calories in beans.[10]

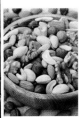

NUTS AND SEEDS

Despite their high-fat content, nuts actually promote weight loss, are low in glycemic load, protect against heart disease, and have anti-inflammatory effects that may prevent insulin resistance.[11]

LOW-SUGAR FRESH FRUIT

Stick with low-sugar fruits such as berries, kiwi, oranges, pomegranate, and melon to minimize glycemic effects.

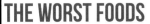

THE WORST FOODS

These foods elevate blood glucose levels, reduce insulin sensitivity and elevate the risk for type 2 diabetes. Sadly, they are also the most common foods in our standard American diet.

ADDED SUGARS

Sugar-sweetened beverages, fruit juices, honey, maple syrup, sugary processed foods, and desserts promote hyperglycemia and insulin resistance.[12]

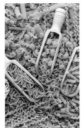

REFINED GRAINS

Refined carbs like white rice, white pasta, and white bread are missing fiber, so they raise blood glucose levels high and fast. In addition, cooked starchy foods also contain by-products that promote aging and diabetes complications.[12, 13]

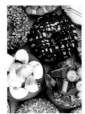

FRIED FOODS

Potato chips, French fries, doughnuts, and other fried starches are high-glycemic, high-calorie and low-nutrient foods which, because they are cooked at high temperatures, contain harmful byproducts.[14]

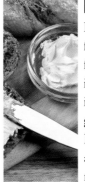

MARGARINE AND BUTTER

High-saturated fat, refined oil based foods such as margarine, shortening, fast food and processed baked goods increase cardiovascular risk and reduce insulin sensitivity, leading to elevated glucose and insulin levels.[15]
Even using non-trans-fat margarines and real butter regularly increase insulin resistance, making it almost impossible to control your diabetes.

RED AND PROCESSED MEATS

Several studies with large numbers of participants confirm that the consumption of meat increases the risk of diabetes and premature death.[3]

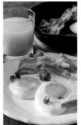

EGGS

There are clear links between eating eggs and an increased risk for diabetes and for cardiovascular disease in people who already have diabetes.. Eggs and diabetes are not a good mix; they increase the risk of death in diabetics. [16-18]

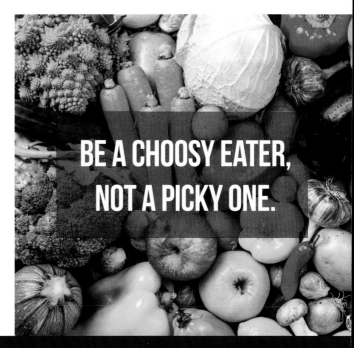

BE A CHOOSY EATER, NOT A PICKY ONE.

THE IMPORTANCE OF GLYCEMIC LOAD

WHAT IS GLYCEMIC LOAD?

Glycemic load is a term used to describe the ability of a food to raise blood glucose (sugar).

Carbohydrates are complex sugar molecules in foods that the body breaks down into its simplest form, called glucose. The composition of the food determines how easily the carbohydrates are digested and absorbed into the bloodstream.

WHAT IS GLYCEMIC INDEX?

Since not all carbohydrates are digested or absorbed at the same rate, the glycemic index (GI) is a relative ranking of carbohydrate in foods according to how they affect blood glucose levels. Foods whose sugar molecules enter the bloodstream more slowly have a lower GI than foods whose sugar molecules enter the bloodstream more quickly. Low GI foods are more slowly digested, absorbed and metabolized, and cause a lower and slower rise in blood glucose and, therefore, insulin levels. Foods that contain large amounts of fiber, resistant starch, and slowly digestible starch have low GIs, as they take a longer time to be absorbed.

THE IMPORTANCE OF GLYCEMIC LOAD

Knowing the glycemic load of a certain food is a more valuable marker for those with diabetes than knowing a food's glycemic index. That's because glycemic load is a measure of both the quality (the GI value) and the quantity (grams per serving) of a carbohydrate in a meal. It's the more practical number because it considers the amount of food eaten in a serving as well as how fast the sugar in the meal will enter the bloodstream. A food's glycemic load is determined by multiplying its glycemic index by the amount of carbohydrate the food contains in each serving and dividing by 100. GL is a useful number for comparing typical serving sizes of different foods.

THE GLYCEMIC LOAD OF COMMON FOODS

This table makes it easy to understand why I recommend using beans as the major carbohydrate source – instead of potatoes, bread, white rice, and pasta.

FOOD (SERVING SIZE)	GLYCEMIC LOAD (GL) [19]
HIGH GL FOODS: 20 or greater	
White potato (1 medium baked)	29
White rice (1 cup cooked)	26
White pasta (1 cup cooked)	24
White flour bagel (1, 3.5-inch diameter)	24
Chocolate cake (1/10 box cake mix + 2T frosting)	20
White bread (2 slices)	20
INTERMEDIATE GL FOODS: 11-19	
Raisins (1/4 cup)	19
Corn (1 cup cooked)	18
Whole wheat bread (2 slices)	18
Black rice (1 cup cooked)	15
Grapes (1 cup)	14
Sweet potato (1 medium baked)	14
Rolled oats (1 cup cooked)	13
Mango (1 cup)	11
Whole wheat berries/kernels (1 cup cooked)	11
LOW GL FOODS: 10 or less	
Lentils (1 cup)	9
Apple (1 medium)	9
Kiwi (2 medium)	9
Green peas (1 cup cooked)	8
Butternut squash (1 cup cooked)	8
Kidney beans (1 cup)	7
Blueberries (1 cup)	7
Black beans (1 cup)	6
Watermelon (1 cup)	6
Orange (1 medium)	4
Carrots (1 cup cooked)	3
Carrots (1 cup raw)	2
Cashews (1 ounce)	2
Strawberries (1 cup)	1
Other nuts and seeds	Negligible
Cauliflower	Negligible
Eggplant	Negligible
Tomatoes	Negligible
Mushrooms	Negligible
Onions	Negligible

FREQUENTLY ASKED QUESTIONS

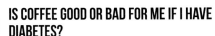

IS COFFEE GOOD OR BAD FOR ME IF I HAVE DIABETES?

The research on coffee is still unclear. Caffeine in the short term is known to impair insulin sensitivity (the body's normal response to insulin) and increase blood glucose.[20] However, some studies have actually linked coffee drinking to a lower risk of diabetes.[21] This may be because the antioxidants in coffee provide some benefits, especially to people eating an overall low-antioxidant diet. For all people, caffeine is problematic because it is a stimulant. It allows you to get by on inadequate sleep and often increases appetite, which might hinder weight loss. Drinking one cup of coffee a day most likely will not interfere with your health goals, but if you rely on several cups a day to keep you awake, what you really need is sleep.

HOW DO I EAT AT A RESTAURANT ON THIS PLAN?

Dining out can be challenging, but works well when you plan ahead. Check menus ahead of time, and find restaurants that have healthful options. For breakfast, most places will have oatmeal and fresh fruit. For lunch and dinner, scan the menu for large, entree-size salads. Ask for the dressing on the side and use only a small amount, or ask for lemon juice or vinegar instead. Look at a restaurant's side dishes for what vegetables they offer; include the vegetables that are offered with their animal-product meals. Then, pick the ones you like the most and request a meal out of them. Always stress not to add salt and, if possible, no oil. After doing some research and trying places out, you will get to know the restaurants in your area that will accommodate your dietary needs.

DOES VINEGAR REDUCE BLOOD SUGAR?

Yes. Consuming vinegar with a meal has been shown to reduce the increase in blood glucose after the meal.[22] Use vinegar in your salad dressings to get this benefit at lunch and dinner.

FRUIT HAS SUGAR. SHOULDN'T I AVOID IT?

Naturally sweet fruits aren't off-limits – they provide many valuable phytochemicals. In fact, higher fresh fruit intake is associated with a lower risk of type 2 diabetes.[23]

However, there are guidelines:

1. Most often choose fruits that are lower in sugar and have plenty of fiber to slow the absorption of that sugar; these include berries, pomegranate, kiwi, oranges, tart apples and melon.

2. Limit fruit to five servings daily, one of which should be some type of berries.

DOES THE *TRANSFORMATION 20 DIABETES PLAN* HAVE TO BE ALL OR NOTHING?

No, but the benefits you get out of this plan will be proportional to the effort you put in. If you follow the plan half the time, you can expect only half the benefit. From my more than 25 years of experience with patients, I have concluded that it is much more difficult to do this program 80 or 90 percent of the time because the constant decision-making is stressful. When you go all the way and make a full commitment, it is so much easier, and the results are miraculous.

WILL I BE HUNGRY?

You will probably feel unwell at first, as your body's detoxification processes are working. I call this experience toxic hunger, and it will usually disappear within the first week. It is analogous to withdrawal from caffeine, and the physical feelings include lightheadedness, fatigue, headaches, shakiness and irritability.

While detoxing, you may also have some digestive discomfort, such as bloating or gas, as your body adjusts to this high-fiber diet. You can minimize the discomfort by chewing better, and eating beans in smaller amounts (adding more over time), and, in the beginning, eating more vegetables cooked and a smaller amount raw. Gradually increase the raw vegetable portions and decrease the cooked amount.

IF I SLIP UP ONE DAY, SHOULD I START OVER FROM THE BEGINNING OR PICK UP WHERE I LEFT OFF?

Pick up where you left off. The most important thing is not to let one off day derail you from your goals.

HOW CAN I DO THIS PLAN IF I DON'T HAVE ENOUGH TIME TO COOK?

Nutritarian meals can be quick and easy when you are busy, or complex gourmet cuisine when you have the time to spend in the kitchen. These recipes and meal plans are examples of some great-tasting meals, but you can keep to the Transformation 20 guidelines and make simpler meals. One of the simplest Nutritarian meals is raw vegetables dipped in low-salt hummus. For another quick meal, top prewashed mixed greens with shredded cabbage or cut-up broccoli and canned beans. Then, mash (with a fork) a bit of nut butter with a flavored vinegar or lemon juice and mix until creamy and use this as the dressing to the salad. Finish the meal with a piece of fruit, or cut up the fruit and add it to the salad. I also produce and sell some healthy sauces and dressings that make eating like a gourmet simple and fast. You put some vegetables in a wok or pot, add some of the flavorful sauce, heat and stir, and that's it.

IS CONTROLLING MY BLOOD SUGAR WITH DIET REALLY DIFFERENT FROM CONTROLLING IT WITH MEDICATION?

Yes. Just lowering blood sugar with medication does not curtail the damage. If you don't change your diet, your diabetes will more than likely get worse with worsening complications. To stop the damage that diabetes causes, your weight has to normalize and your insulin resistance has to improve. Many of the underlying causes of diabetic complications, which are the same underlying causes of heart disease and cancer, will continue. Like almost all heart disease and most cancers, type 2 diabetes is a food-borne illness, and the only way to discontinue the harm it causes is by stopping what caused it in the first place. By addressing diabetes with a Nutritarian diet, you not only control your blood glucose, you ingest anti-cancer compounds, prevent or counteract oxidative damage, produce more anti-inflammatory compounds, reduce blood pressure and cholesterol, and improve your overall health. For most type 2 diabetics, this means no more medication is needed as blood sugar is normalized, and for type 1 diabetics, less insulin is needed and that, in turn, produces a more stable blood sugar, minimizing highs and lows.

WON'T A GLASS OF WINE EVERY DAY BE GOOD FOR MY HEART?

Although there have been studies that show wine having some health benefits, that would only be for the person eating the unhealthful Standard American diet. For example, alcohol interferes with the body's blood-clotting mechanisms, and this is only a benefit in those who have an abnormally high risk of clotting from eating unhealthfully.[24] Although red wine does contain some flavonoids and the antioxidant resveratrol, adding alcoholic beverages to a healthful, antioxidant-rich diet will not provide any further benefit. It's also important to know that even light drinking is linked to an increased risk of cancer.[25] Plus, liquid calories are unfavorable for diabetes. So in a nutshell, I do not recommend drinking a glass of wine every day for a person eating a Nutritarian diet.

NO OLIVE OIL?

Nuts and seeds are better fat sources, because they are whole foods. The fiber in nuts and seeds slows the absorption of calories, and binds cholesterol for removal in the stool. All oils promote weight gain, whereas nuts are known to help maintain a healthy weight.[26] The health benefits of the Mediterranean diet are often mistakenly attributed to olive oil instead of the abundance of unrefined plant foods, like vegetables, fruits, nuts, beans, and grains. Though a diet with oil, such as the Mediterranean diet, may be a step in the right direction, and be somewhat better than the Standard American diet, it still does not reverse diabetes or lower blood pressure and body weight like a Nutritarian diet will. Oil is fattening and promotes diabetes, and can sabotage your success.

MINIMIZE SALT TO WHAT LEVEL?

All foods contain natural sodium, and the level contained in natural foods is sufficient for our needs. Excess sodium elevates blood pressure; it stiffens the arteries over time and increases the risk of heart disease and stroke.[27] It will take time to retrain taste buds that are accustomed to a high-salt diet. To add flavor, try spicing up your meals with gourmet vinegars, herbs, spices, no-salt seasoning mixes, cayenne pepper or hot pepper flakes. Try not to allow more than a few hundred milligrams of sodium each day, over and above the sodium contained in natural foods.

DO I NEED TO COUNT CARBOHYDRATES?

No. Some physicians recommend their diabetic patients design their diet around staying below a specific number of grams of carbohydrate each day. The carbohydrate count is an incomplete picture – it doesn't tell you how the food affects blood glucose (see page 7 for a table of high- and low-glycemic carbohydrate sources). The calories in a Nutritarian diabetes reversal diet come mainly from low-glycemic, high-fiber, high-nutrient carbohydrate foods, such as beans, peas, greens and berries; plus healthful fat sources, like nuts and seeds. When using these caloric sources that are absorbed more slowly than bread, white rice and potato, you need not count carbs and you will see dramatic benefits on reducing body fat, insulin resistance and blood glucose. Of course, it is important not to overeat, even on healthful foods.

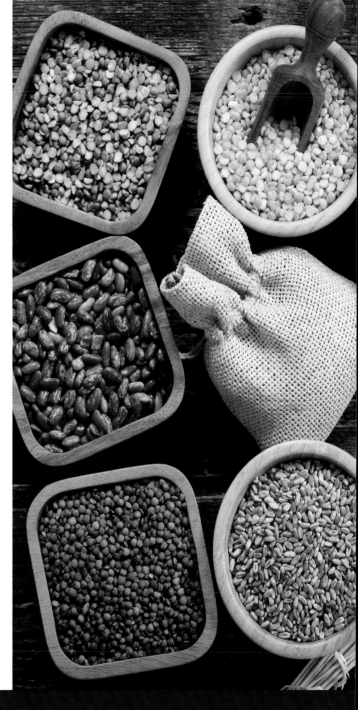

IMPORTANT SUPPLEMENTS

OMEGA-3 DHA AND EPA: These fats help to maintain brain health, starting from development and into old age.[36] I recommend algae-derived, lab grown vegan DHA and EPA as it has no pollutants and is more sustainable than fish oil.

DO NOT TAKE THESE SUPPLEMENTS

These nutrients, when taken as supplements, have been shown to be harmful. When shopping for a multivitamin, avoid ones that include these ingredients:[37-41]

- Beta-carotene
- Vitamin A
- Vitamin E
- Folic acid
- Copper

THE VITAMINS AND MINERALS IMPORTANT TO SUPPLEMENT

VITAMIN D: The primary source of vitamin D is the sun, and insufficiency is common. Low vitamin D levels are linked to osteoporosis, cardiovascular disease, depression, autoimmune disease, cancer and diabetes.[28] Supplement to keep vitamin D blood levels between 30 and 45 ng/ml.

VITAMIN K2: A Nutritarian diet provides plenty of vitamin K1, but vitamin K2 is low in plant foods. I recommend taking supplemental K2 for bone and cardiovascular health.[29, 30]

VITAMIN B12: This vitamin is not present in plant foods, and our absorption becomes less efficient as we age. B12 is important for brain function, red blood cell production, and DNA synthesis.[31]

IODINE: Iodine is needed to produce thyroid hormones, and the main source is iodized salt. On a Nutritarian diet, you will be minimizing salt, so I recommend taking supplemental iodine.[32]

ZINC: Getting enough zinc is important for immune function and hundreds of chemical reactions throughout the body.[33, 34] Though too much supplemental zinc can be unfavorable, the absorption of zinc decreases with age, and supplementation has been shown to decrease the risk of pneumonia in the elderly.[35]

VITAMINS AND MINERALS SPECIFICALLY IMPORTANT FOR DIABETICS

THIAMIN: People with diabetes are at risk of excreting too much thiamin, resulting in deficiency. Thiamin (vitamin B1) is involved in glucose metabolism and insulin production, and over time, thiamin deficiency may lead to a greater risk of diabetes complications. [42, 43] I recommend that people with diabetes take some extra thiamin — a conservative dose of approximately 10 mg — along with a Nutritarian diet.

CHROMIUM: The essential mineral chromium is also important for producing energy from glucose, and people with diabetes are more likely to have low chromium levels. High-dose chromium supplements have been found to reduce fasting blood glucose.[44, 45] However, a modest dose plus a Nutritarian diet will provide adequate chromium. I recommend using chromium picolinate, which is more absorbable than other forms of chromium,[46] and a conservative dose of 40 mcg.

HELPFUL SUPPLEMENTS FOR DIABETICS WHEN STARTING THE PROGRAM

Once you have your blood glucose under good control with a Nutritarian lifestyle, the supplements below will likely not provide further benefit. Always keep in mind: Diet and exercise are the most important parts of this program.

CINNAMON: Supplemental cinnamon powder and cinnamon extracts have been shown in numerous studies to reduce fasting blood glucose in diabetics.[47, 48] The most common type of cinnamon, Cassia, contains coumarin (Ceylon cinnamon does not), a substance which may damage the liver. Therefore, for the safest cinnamon, I recommend using Ceylon cinnamon. Purified cinnamon extracts are also available as supplements.

GREEN TEA: Green tea contains antioxidants such as EGCG that are very rare in other plant foods. Drinking brewed green tea regularly has been associated with a lower risk of type 2 diabetes and cardiovascular disease. A meta-analysis of (17 total) trials using green tea extract as a supplement concluded that green tea extract reduced fasting blood glucose and HbA1c (a long-term indicator of blood glucose levels).[49, 50]

ALOE VERA: Aloe vera gel – the plant's stored water source – contains vitamins, minerals, plant sterols, antioxidants and anti-inflammatory compounds, and has been studied for its effects on blood glucose. A few studies on people with either diabetes or prediabetes supplementing with aloe vera gel powder found decreases in fasting blood glucose.[51]

OTHER PLANT EXTRACTS: White mulberry leaf, banaba leaf, gymnema leaf, and fenugreek seed phytochemicals in preliminary human studies have helped to limit elevations in blood glucose after a meal.[52-55]

Most of Dr. Fuhrman's diabetic patients take this effective and convenient combination of supplements to aid their health and protect against diabetes:

DHA-EPA Purity

Glucose Biotect

LDL Biotect

Women's Daily Formula + D3

Men's Daily Formula +D3

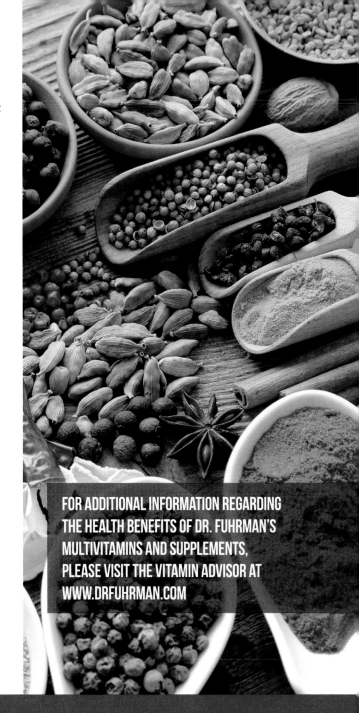

FOR ADDITIONAL INFORMATION REGARDING THE HEALTH BENEFITS OF DR. FUHRMAN'S MULTIVITAMINS AND SUPPLEMENTS, PLEASE VISIT THE VITAMIN ADVISOR AT WWW.DRFUHRMAN.COM

GET MOVING

Performing daily exercise and building up your exercise tolerance are among the most effective ways to enhance your recovery from diabetes. The more out of shape you are, the more trouble you will have doing much exercise, and the more frequently you'll have to exercise. Engage in regular but shorter periods of exercise. Remember short periods of exercise add up. So even if you cannot sustain an extended period of exercise, you can still get huge benefits, by staying upright, moving around, and performing exercises throughout the day for three to five minutes.

One way to look at exercise is to consider it a debt to be paid. Eat your next meal only after you have exercised to work up an appetite. Exercise is excellent medicine: it helps keep blood glucose down, improves the health of the heart and the brain, and it's a natural way to improve your mood. A good place to start is by walking. Then,

get to a point while walking that you pick your knees up as high as possible. Try it for five or 10 minutes, three or more times a day. Short intervals make exercise easy to fit into a busy life and allow you to quickly build up stamina over a short period of time.

TAKE EVERY OPPORTUNITY TO GET FIT

Walking up flights of stairs is the best exercise. Walk up as many stairs as you can each day. I often tell my patients to walk up and down the stairs five times in the morning, five times before lunch and five times each night. It only takes five minutes, but it works.

Remember, weight loss is mostly what you eat (or don't eat); you can't out-exercise your mouth. In other words, exercise cannot balance eating poorly. But increasing your strength and muscle mass through weight training

and weight-bearing exercises helps to metabolize more calories and improve your fat-to-muscle ratio. By increasing muscle density, you will help normalize your metabolism and that, in turn, will help address the problem that's causing diabetes.

I also encourage patients to join a health club and use a variety of equipment to focus on different body parts for maximum results.

EVEN LIGHT ACTIVITY MAKES A DIFFERENCE

Some people have health conditions that preclude them from vigorous exercise. However, that does not let you off the hook. An exercise prescription can be devised to fit even limited capabilities. Almost everyone can do something. Start slow and gradually build up to your level of tolerance so you don't injure yourself.

- Take the stairs instead of the elevator
- Park your car away from stores or buildings You visit
- Take an extra lap around the grocery store
- Take a walking meeting
- Avoid sitting when you can
- Put the computer on a counter to stand while you type
- Walk while you talk on the phone
- Dance like no one is watching
- Can't walk? do arm, abdominal and back exercises with light weights
- Bounce up and down in place to music

THE
GROUND RULES

BEFORE YOU GET STARTED . . .

You can anticipate your blood sugar falling with this diet and lifestyle plan. Prevent the occurrence of hypoglycemic episodes by maintaining good communication with your physician and careful monitoring of blood sugar levels.

If you are hungry, at meal times eat more of the foods you can eat liberally: raw vegetables, cooked non-starchy vegetables, and beans. But, try very hard not to eat even these foods between mealtimes, and resist the urge to eat recreationally, or when you are not truly hungry. You can also eat larger portions or an extra portion of menu items that contain only these foods.

Refer to the next page for the chart of Foods to Eat Liberally, Eat in Moderation or Avoid Entirely

The *Transformation 20* is based on eating large quantities of raw and cooked vegetables. These foods fill you up and leave little room for processed, refined foods, which contain lots of calories but few nutrients. Nutrient-dense vegetables are the most important foods to focus on for diabetes prevention and reversal. Aim for between a half and a full pound of raw vegetables, and the same amount of cooked vegetables, each day. To give you a general idea, a pound of raw vegetables is a salad composed of: 5 cups of chopped romaine lettuce, 1 cup of shredded cabbage, 1 medium tomato, 1 small carrot and ¼ cup chopped raw onion. For cooked portions, 1 ½ cups of broccoli is about 8 ounces and 1 ½ cups of kale weighs 7 ounces. You can eat as much as you want of greens and raw salad vegetables, but do not eat until distended or uncomfortable, and try to stop eating before feeling full.

Beans, lentils and other legumes are the ideal carbohydrate source, with low glycemic load due to their protein, fiber and resistant starch. While fiber and resistant starch are classified as carbohydrates, they are not broken down in the small intestine, which reduces the amount of calories that are absorbed.

Fruit is a good choice for satisfying sweet cravings. Fruits are rich in fiber and antioxidants. Berries, kiwi, oranges and melon are low-sugar fruits that are included in many of the *Transformation 20* menus.

Lunch and dinner recipes are interchangeable, so feel free to swap meals within these categories or repeat a meal more often than it is on the menu. When you have leftovers, they can be substituted for other meals. If you like a recipe, double it and freeze it in individual portions so you don't have to do as much cooking. Just don't have a meal that contains bread more than three times a week, and don't have a breakfast meal more than once a day. Recipes that include animal products should also be limited to three times per week.

Frozen vegetables and fruit can be substituted for fresh. Don't use canned vegetables or fruit. Canned products lose nutrients during processing, and often contain added sugar or salt.

As you change your diet and discontinue unhealthy, addictive foods, your body may go through a detox or withdrawal phase where you feel weak or uncomfortable, or experience headaches or cravings for certain foods. This means that your body is healing, and the removal of toxins is underway. These symptoms will start to resolve gradually as you flood your body with high-nutrient, whole plant foods. The discomfort rarely continues after the first week.

Your stomach doesn't have teeth. Chew your food very well, until it feels liquefied in your mouth before swallowing. It takes the digestive tract time to adjust to a high-fiber diet that contains lots of raw vegetables and beans. Chewing well will help ease the digestive process, and also ensures that more nutrients are available for absorption.

FOODS TO EAT LIBERALLY, EAT IN MODERATION OR
AVOID ENTIRELY

Whether you want to lose weight or just eat more healthfully, an easy way to make the right dietary choices is to sort foods into three categories: those you may eat liberally, those you should eat in moderation, or those you should avoid entirely. Note that the term "eat liberally" is more accurate than the term "unlimited." Unlimited could imply overeating, or recreational or emotional eating, or eating when not hungry. Also, consuming too much of a very healthy food, such as fruit, can lead to insufficient vegetables in your diet.

FOLLOW THESE GUIDELINES:

EAT LIBERALLY
You can eat as much as you want of these foods: (within reason):
- **Raw vegetables** (*Goal: about ½ to 1 pound daily*)
- **Cooked green and non-green nutrient–dense vegetables** (*Goal: about ½ to 1 pound daily*)
  Non-green nutrient dense veggies are: tomatoes, cauliflower, eggplant, mushrooms, peppers, onions and carrots
- **Beans, legumes, tofu, lentils, tempeh and edamame** (*Goal: ½-1 cup daily*)
- **Fresh or frozen fruit** (3 to 5 per day; 1 serving = 1 piece or 1 to 1 1/2 cups berries or chopped fruit)

EAT IN MODERATION
Include these foods in your diet, but limit the amount you are eating:
- **Cooked starchy vegetables or whole grains** (*Maximum: 2 servings daily; 1 serving = 1 cup or 1 slice*)
  - Butternut and other winter squashes
  - Sweet potatoes (*avoid white potatoes*)
  - Corn, quinoa, farro, or other intact whole grains
  - 100% whole grain bread
- **Raw nuts and seeds.** (Eat at least 1 ounce or 1/4 cup per day; Limit to a maximum of 2 ounces for women or 3 ounces for men)
- **Avocado** (*Maximum ½ per day*)
- **Dried Fruit** (*Maximum 2 tablespoons per day*)
- **Animal Products: fat-free dairy, clean wild fish and certified organic poultry** (*Maximum of 6 ounces per week, limit each serving size to 2 ounces and use as a minor component/flavoring agent*)

Note: If you are not trying to lose weight, amounts of cooked starchy vegetables, intact whole grains, nuts, seeds, and avocado may be moderately increased depending on your caloric needs.

AVOID ENTIRELY
Do not consume any of the following:
- **Products made with sugar or white flour**
- **Soda and soft drinks** (including those made with artificial sweeteners)
- **Fruit Juice**
- **Barbequed, processed and cured meats and all red meat**
- **Full-fat and reduced-fat dairy** (*cheese, icecream, butter, milk*)
- **Eggs**
- **All vegetable oils,** (*including olive oil and coconut oil*)

Note: If you are not trying to lose weight, a small amount of olive oil, a teaspoon a day or less may be used.

STOCK YOUR PANTRY

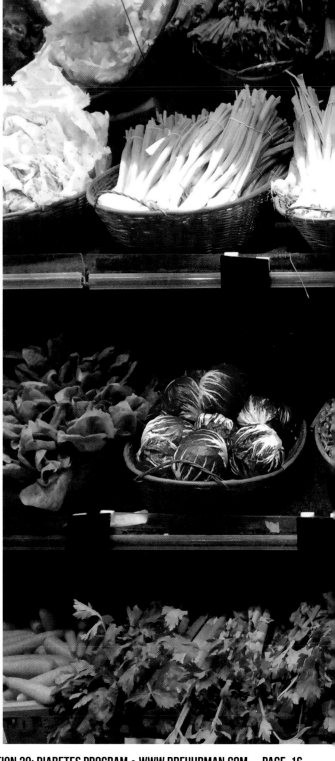

Before you begin the meal plan, clean out your refrigerator and cabinets of all trigger foods or designate a space for your healthy foods. Stock your pantry with these staple items. They will be needed for the recipes and meals you will be preparing for the next 20 days. Four additional shopping lists are also included with the menus. These are compiled for five-day periods and include perishable items and other foods specific to each set of menus.

NUTS AND SEEDS
All nuts and seeds should be raw and unsalted

Walnuts

Cashews

Almonds

Chia seeds

Hemp seeds

Flax seeds

Unhulled sesame seeds

Pumpkin seeds

Sunflower seeds

Raw almond butter

Natural unsalted peanut butter

DRIED HERBS AND SPICES
No-salt seasoning blend such as
 Dr. Fuhrman's VegiZest or Mrs. Dash

No-salt seasoning blend such as
 Dr. Fuhrman's MatoZest or Italian seasoning blend

Cajun or other spicy seasoning blend

Garlic powder

Onion powder

Dried oregano

Dried basil

Thyme

Rosemary

Black pepper

Chili powder

Curry powder

Red curry powder

Cumin

Coriander

Turmeric

Crushed red pepper flakes

Bay leaf

Dry mustard powder

Cinnamon

Nutmeg

Alcohol-free vanilla extract

WHOLE GRAINS, DRIED FRUIT, VINEGARS AND OTHER ITEMS
Old-fashioned rolled oats and steel-cut oats

Buckwheat groats

Quinoa

Farro

Wild rice

100% whole-grain flour tortillas, such as
 Ezekiel or Alvarado Street brands (store
 in freezer)

100% whole-grain pitas, such as Ezekiel or
 Alvarado Street brands (store in freezer)

Rice vinegar

White wine vinegar

Balsamic vinegar

Bragg Liquid Aminos or low-sodium
 soy sauce

Nutritional yeast

Dijon mustard

Dates

Raisins

Unsweetened dried coconut

Natural non-alkalized cocoa powder

Cornmeal

DAYS 1-5
SHOPPING LIST

This shopping list assumes that all recipes in the meal plan will be made. Menus frequently include fruit for dessert and will mention a specific fruit as an example. That fruit is used for the shopping list.

Make sure you also have all the items listed in the Stock Your Pantry list.

FRESH PRODUCE

VEGETABLES

- [ ] 13 ounces mixed salad greens (13 cups)
- [ ] 2 heads romaine lettuce
- [ ] 5 ounces chopped kale (8 cups)
- [ ] 10 ounces chopped kale, collards or other greens
- [ ] Small head of red cabbage
- [ ] Head of cauliflower
- [ ] Head of broccoli (need 5 cups florets)
- [ ] Your choice of a green vegetable to equal 2 cups cooked (could also buy frozen)
- [ ] 2 red bell peppers
- [ ] 2 green bell peppers
- [ ] Snow peas (need 1 cup)
- [ ] 1 butternut squash (need 3 cups chopped)
- [ ] 1 Portobello mushroom
- [ ] Shiitake mushrooms (need 1 cup sliced)
- [ ] 6 medium tomatoes
- [ ] Pint cherry tomatoes

- [ ] 2 avocados
- [ ] Celery (need 1 stalk)
- [ ] 3 carrots
- [ ] 2 bulbs garlic
- [ ] 4 yellow onions
- [ ] 2 red onions
- [ ] Ginger
- [ ] Parsley
- [ ] Dill

FRUIT

- [ ] 2 ½ cups blueberries (could also use frozen)
- [ ] 2 ½ cups strawberries (could also use frozen)
- [ ] 1 cantaloupe
- [ ] 2 apples
- [ ] 2 navel oranges
- [ ] 2 kiwi
- [ ] 3 bananas
- [ ] 2 lemons
- [ ] 1 lime

REFRIGERATED

- [ ] 2 ½ cups unsweetened, unflavored soy, hemp or almond milk
- [ ] 7 ounces extra-firm tofu
- [ ] Shrimp or chicken (to yield 4 ounces cooked), optional
- [ ] 2 cups carrot juice

FROZEN

This list does not include vegetables and fruit listed under fresh produce that have a frozen option.

- [ ] Green peas (need ⅓ cup)

SHELF STABLE

BEANS

It is assumed that canned low-sodium or no-salt-added beans will be used. If you opt to start with dry beans, 1 cup of dry beans will yield about 3 cups of cooked beans

- [ ] 2 (15 ounce) cans cannellini beans
- [ ] 1 (15 ounce) can chick peas
- [ ] 2 (15 ounce) cans black beans
- [ ] Dry lentils (need 1 cup)
- [ ] Shelled edamame (need 1 cup; could substitute other beans)

OTHER

Choose tomato products packaged in BPA-free materials.

- [ ] 6 ounces firm, lite silken tofu (sold in shelf-stable aseptic boxes)
- [ ] 3 (32 ounce) cartons no-salt-added or low-sodium vegetable broth (need about 10 cups)
- [ ] Kelp powder (need ½ teaspoon)
- [ ] Low-sodium tomato juice (need 1 ⅓ cups)
- [ ] Low-sodium tomato sauce (need ⅔ cup)

DAY 1

Don't live with your diabetes, don't simply control your diabetes — get rid of it.

BREAKFAST

NO-COOK STRAWBERRY OATMEAL
1 SERVING

⅓ cup old-fashioned rolled oats
1 tablespoon chia seeds
⅔ cup unsweetened soy, hemp or almond milk
1 cup fresh or thawed frozen strawberries, sliced (or blueberries, cherries or sliced peaches)
2 tablespoons chopped walnuts

Combine the oats, chia seeds and non-dairy milk. Soak for at least 30 minutes or overnight. Stir in sliced strawberries and walnuts.

CALORIES 334; PROTEIN 13g; CARBOHYDRATES 39g; SUGARS 9g; TOTAL FAT 16g; SATURATED FAT 1.8g; SODIUM 64mg; FIBER 11g

LUNCH

CITRUS SALAD WITH ORANGE SESAME DRESSING
SALAD: 1 SERVING; DRESSING: 3 SERVINGS

For the Orange Sesame Dressing:
1 navel orange, peeled
¼ cup raw cashews
¼ cup hemp seeds
2 tablespoons lightly toasted unhulled sesame seeds
2 tablespoons rice vinegar
½ teaspoon Bragg Liquid Aminos or low-sodium soy sauce
¼ inch piece fresh ginger, peeled
1 clove garlic, chopped

For the Salad:
5 cups mixed baby greens
⅓ ripe avocado, peeled, pitted and sliced

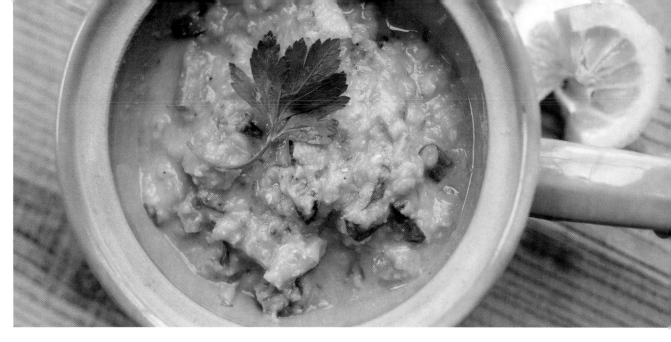

½ navel orange, sliced into rounds
¼ cup thinly sliced red onion

Blend all dressing ingredients in high-powered blender until smooth

To prepare salad, arrange avocado slices, orange rounds and onions on top of lettuce. Pour desired amount of dressing (about ⅓ of the recipe) over salad.

CALORIES 398; PROTEIN 14g; CARBOHYDRATES 45g; SUGARS 22g; TOTAL FAT 21g; SATURATED FAT 3g; SODIUM 76mg; FIBER 14g

Refrigerate leftover Orange Sesame Dressing. You can substitute it for any of the other dressings over the next 3-4 days of the meal plan.

DINNER

LEMON LENTIL SOUP
4 SERVINGS

1 ½ cups carrots, peeled and chopped
1 cup celery, chopped
4 cups no-salt-added or low-sodium vegetable broth
1 cup dry red lentils, rinsed
¾ teaspoon ground coriander
1 teaspoon ground cumin

3 tablespoons raw cashews
¼ cup fresh lemon juice (about 1 large lemon)
2 cups chopped kale
black pepper, to taste

Place carrots, celery, vegetable broth, lentils, coriander and cumin in a pot and bring to a boil. Reduce heat, cover and simmer for forty minutes or until lentils and vegetables are tender.

In a blender or food processor, blend 1 cup of the soup with cashews and lemon juice. Return to pot along with kale and heat until greens are wilted. Season with black pepper.

CALORIES 289; PROTEIN 20g; CARBOHYDRATES 44g; SUGARS 7g; TOTAL FAT 5.3g; SATURATED FAT 1.1g; SODIUM 144mg; FIBER 17.5g

Men: Have 2 servings of Lemon Lentil Soup.

Portion leftover Lemon Lentil Soup into individual containers. If you are short on time, use it as an alternate lunch or dinner over the next few days or freeze for later use.

Your choice of a cooked green vegetable (can be fresh or frozen).

Tip: Steam or water sauté fresh vegetables. If desired, sauté with fresh chopped garlic or onion. Season with lemon, balsamic vinegar and/or your choice of herbs, spices or a no-salt seasoning blend. For some heat, add red pepper flakes, cayenne pepper or black pepper.

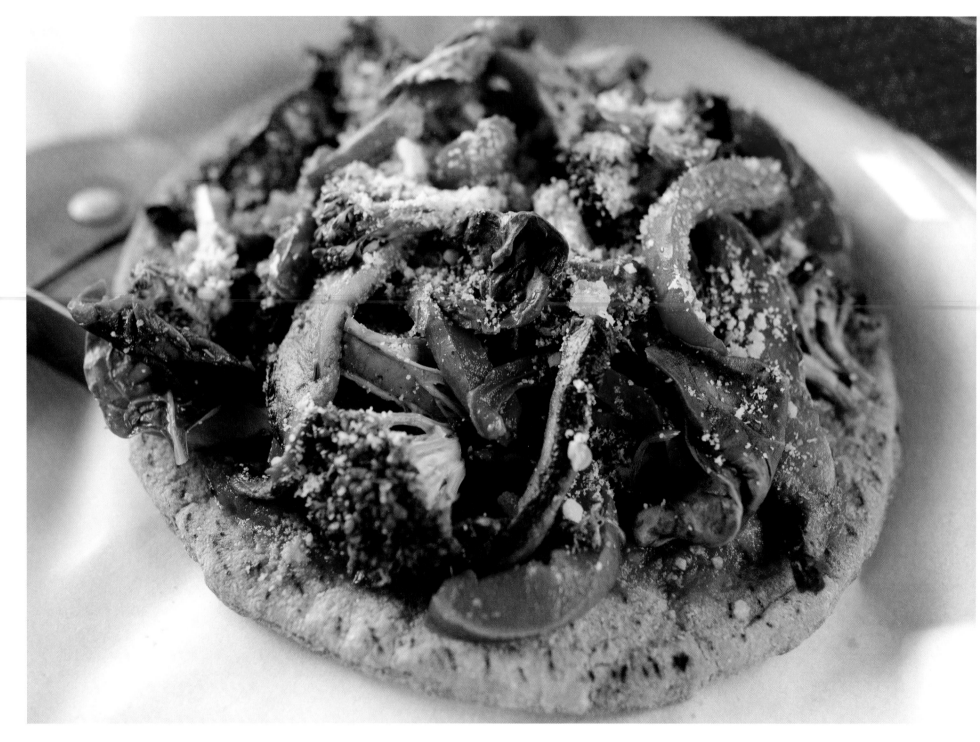

DAY 2

More than 85 percent of the Standard American Diet consists of low-nutrient, high-calorie processed foods, animal foods, dairy products and sweets. These all contribute to excessive weight, high cholesterol and high blood pressure, as well as an epidemic of diabetes.

BREAKFAST

BERRY BOWL
1 SERVING

1 cup fresh or thawed frozen blueberries (or other berries)
1 banana, sliced
¼ cup unsweetened soy, hemp or almond milk
2 tablespoons chopped walnuts or raw almonds
1 tablespoon ground flax seeds or chia seeds

Top berries and banana with non-dairy milk and sprinkle with the nuts and seeds.

CALORIES 317; PROTEIN 6g; CARBOHYDRATES 49g; SUGARS 27g; TOTAL FAT 14g; SATURATED FAT 1.3g; SODIUM 51mg; FIBER 9.1g

Men: Increase chopped walnuts to ¼ cup

> **Tip:** Frozen fruit and vegetables are convenient options. They are rich in micronutrients because they are picked ripe and flash-frozen soon after picking. It is fine to substitute frozen fruit or vegetables for fresh.

LUNCH

QUICK AND EASY BEAN SALAD (or leftover Lemon Lentil Soup from Day 1 dinner with raw veggies dipped in leftover Orange Sesame Dressing from Day 1 lunch)
1 SERVING

1 cup cooked cannellini beans
¼ cup chopped red onion
1 small tomato, chopped
2 tablespoons chopped parsley
1 tablespoon balsamic vinegar
½ teaspoon no-salt seasoning blend such as Dr. Fuhrman's VegiZest or Mrs. Dash
5 cups mixed salad greens

Mix all ingredients except salad greens in a bowl. Serve bean mixture on top of the greens.

CALORIES 364; PROTEIN 25g; CARBOHYDRATES 67g; SUGARS 9g; TOTAL FAT 1.9g; SATURATED FAT 0.4g; SODIUM 131mg; FIBER 19.8g

Men: Mash or slice 1/2 avocado and add to salad

2 kiwi or other fruit for dessert

Leftover cannellini beans can be used for tomorrow's Eat Your Beans Green Smoothie.

> **Tip:** If you use canned beans, choose low-sodium or no-salt-added varieties.

DINNER

ROASTED VEGETABLE PIZZA
1 SERVING

1 cup broccoli florets
½ red bell pepper, sliced
1 Portobello mushroom, cut into ½ inch slices
½ cup halved cherry tomatoes
¼ teaspoon garlic powder
¼ teaspoon onion powder
1 tablespoon balsamic vinegar
1 (100% whole grain) tortilla or pita bread
¼ cup no-salt-added or low-sodium pasta sauce
1-2 tablespoons Nutritarian "Parmesan" (see note)

Preheat oven to 350 degrees F.

Toss broccoli, bell peppers, mushrooms and cherry tomatoes with garlic powder, onion powder and balsamic vinegar. Roast vegetables on a cookie sheet for 15-20 minutes or until tender, turning occasionally and mounding to keep from drying out.

Bake tortilla or pita directly on oven rack for 4 minutes or just until slightly crisp. Spread a thin layer of pasta sauce on tortilla or on top of pita bread, and distribute roasted vegetables on top. Sprinkle with Nutritarian Parmesan. Bake for an additional 3-4 minutes, checking occasionally to avoid browning.

Note: To make Nutritarian Parmesan, place ¼ cup walnuts and ¼ cup nutritional yeast in a food processor and pulse until the texture of grated Parmesan is achieved. Store leftovers in an airtight container and refrigerate. (You can use this as a topping for salads or cooked vegetables. You will also use it again for lunch on Day 11.)

CALORIES 309; PROTEIN 16g; CARBOHYDRATES 45g; SUGARS 10g; TOTAL FAT 8.0g; SATURATED FAT 1.0g; SODIUM 192mg; FIBER 11.3g

Leftover red bell pepper can be used in tomorrow's Chickpea Tuno Salad. If you are following a gluten-free diet, substitute a dinner from another day.

Salad (use romaine lettuce, tomatoes, onions and other veggies) with Easy Balsamic Almond Dressing (or use leftover Orange Sesame Dressing from Day 1 lunch)

EASY BALSAMIC ALMOND DRESSING
1 SERVING

2 tablespoons water
1 tablespoon plus 1 teaspoon balsamic vinegar
1 tablespoon raw almond butter
¼ teaspoon onion powder
¼ teaspoon garlic powder
⅛ teaspoon dried oregano
⅛ teaspoon dried basil

Whisk water, vinegar and almond butter together until mixture is smooth and almond butter is evenly dispersed. Mix in remaining ingredients.

CALORIES 127; PROTEIN 4g; CARBOHYDRATES 9g; SUGARS 5g; TOTAL FAT 9g; SATURATED FAT 0.7g; SODIUM 10mg; FIBER 2g

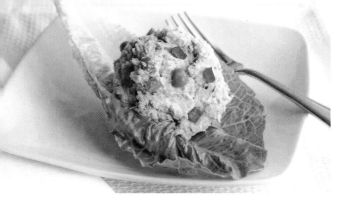

DAY 3

A nutrient-rich menu of green vegetables, berries, beans, mushrooms, onions, seeds and other natural foods is the key to achieving optimal weight and health.

BREAKFAST

EAT YOUR BEANS GREEN SMOOTHIE
1 SERVING

1 ½ cups kale
½ banana (see tip)
½ cup fresh or frozen blueberries
⅓ cup cooked white beans, any variety
½ cup unsweetened soy, hemp or almond milk
¼ cup water
1 tablespoon flax seeds

Blend all ingredients in a high-powered blender until smooth.

CALORIES 282; PROTEIN 12g; CARBOHYDRATES 51g; SUGARS 14; TOTAL FAT 5.9g; SATURATED FAT 0.5g; SODIUM 143mg; FIBER 11.4g

> **Tip:** Freeze leftover banana halves or ripe bananas that you will not get a chance to eat. They will be used in smoothies and frozen desserts.

LUNCH

Chickpea Tuno Salad served with tomato wedges on a bed of chopped romaine lettuce

CHICKPEA TUNO SALAD
3 SERVINGS

1 ½ cups cooked chickpeas or 1 (15 ounce) can no-salt-added or low-sodium chickpeas, drained
¼ cup raw almonds
¼ cup walnuts
1 tablespoon lemon juice, or more to taste
½ teaspoon kelp powder
6 ounces firm lite silken tofu (see note)
1 ½ tablespoons white wine vinegar
¼ teaspoon dry mustard powder
1 tablespoon nutritional yeast
1 ½ teaspoons Dijon mustard
1 medium celery stalk, diced
¼ cup red bell pepper, minced
⅓ cup frozen peas, thawed
freshly ground black pepper

In a food processor, pulse the chickpeas, walnuts and almonds until coarsely chopped. Add the lemon juice and kelp powder and pulse a few more times. Transfer to a large mixing bowl.

Place the tofu, vinegar, dry mustard, nutritional yeast and Dijon mustard in a high-powered blender and blend until very smooth. Add to the mixing bowl with the chickpea mixture, along with the celery, red pepper, peas and black pepper. Mix thoroughly. Cover and refrigerate for at least 30 minutes to let the flavors mingle before serving.

Note: Silken tofu (also called Japanese-style tofu) has a softer consistency than regular tofu. Unlike regular tofu, silken tofu is sometimes packaged in aseptic boxes that do not require refrigeration. Because of this, silken tofu may be sold in a different section of the grocery store than regular tofu which is packed in water and requires refrigeration.

CALORIES 338; PROTEIN 18g; CARBOHYDRATES 32g; SUGARS 7g; TOTAL FAT 17g; SATURATED FAT 1.6g; SODIUM 87mg; FIBER 10g

Refrigerate leftover Chickpea Tuno Salad. It makes a great alternate lunch choice over the next 2-3 days.

Cantaloupe or other fruit for dessert

DINNER

BROCCOLI AND SHIITAKE MUSHROOMS WITH THAI PEANUT SAUCE (with optional chicken or shrimp)
2 SERVINGS

For the Thai Peanut Sauce:
1 cup water
4 regular dates or 2 Medjool dates, pitted
3 tablespoons natural, unsalted peanut butter
1 ½ tablespoons unsweetened shredded coconut
1 teaspoon minced ginger
1 tablespoon lime juice
½ teaspoon red curry powder
½ teaspoon chili powder
½ teaspoon ground cumin

For the Vegetables:
½ cup chopped onions
4 cups broccoli florets
1 cup thinly sliced red bell pepper strips
1 cup trimmed snow peas
1 cup sliced shiitake mushrooms

To make the sauce, blend water and dates in a high-powered blender, then add peanut butter, coconut, ginger, lime juice and spices and blend again until smooth and well-combined.

To cook the vegetables, heat ¼ cup water in a large non-stick wok or skillet, then add chopped onions and broccoli, cover and cook for 4 minutes stirring occasionally and adding additional water as needed to prevent sticking. Remove cover and add red bell pepper strips, shiitake mushrooms and snow peas and cook for an additional 4 minutes or until vegetables are crisp-tender. Add desired amount of sauce and continue to stir fry for 1-2 minutes to heat through.

CALORIES 351; PROTEIN 16g; CARBOHYDRATES 46g; SUGARS 21g; TOTAL FAT 16g; SATURATED FAT 4.2g; SODIUM 94mg; FIBER 14g

Serve with ⅔ cup cooked wild rice per serving. If desired, may be topped with 2 ounces of cooked shrimp or shredded chicken per serving.

> **Tip:** Use water or low-sodium vegetable broth instead of oil to sauté your onions, garlic and other vegetables. Simply heat a skillet on high heat, add 2-3 tablespoons of liquid and when it's hot, add the vegetables. You can cover the pan occasionally to help the food cook faster. Let the pan get dry enough for the food to start to brown just a little before you add more liquid.

DAY 4

Knowledge is the key that can set you free from the vicious cycle of food addiction and self-destructive eating practices. Get rid of the on-a-diet mentality and become an expert in nutritional excellence.

BREAKFAST

BUTTERNUT BLUEBERRY BREAKFAST
2 SERVINGS

3 cups peeled, seeded butternut squash, chopped in ½ inch cubes (see note)

1 medium apple, peeled, cored and cut into pieces

½ teaspoon cinnamon

¼ teaspoon nutmeg

⅓ cup water

1 cup fresh or frozen blueberries

¼ cup chopped walnuts

2 tablespoons raisins

Place squash, apples, cinnamon, nutmeg and water in a sauce-pan. Bring to a boil and reduce heat. Cover and cook until tender, about 15 minutes, adding more water, if needed. Mash with a potato masher, leaving the mixture chunky.

Heat frozen blueberries with walnuts and raisins and stir well. Top mashed butternut squash with blueberry mixture.

Note: To save time, try precut or frozen butternut squash.

CALORIES 297; PROTEIN 5g; CARBOHYDRATES 53g; SUGARS 26g; TOTAL FAT 10g; SATURATED FAT 1.0g; SODIUM 12mg; FIBER 9g

LUNCH

Big Green Salad with Creamy Roasted Garlic Dressing Include mixed greens, romaine, tomatoes, red onions, shredded red cabbage, and edamame or other cooked beans

CREAMY ROASTED GARLIC DRESSING
4 SERVINGS

1 bulb garlic

⅔ cup unsweetened soy, almond or hemp milk

½ cup raw almonds

2 tablespoons raw pumpkin seeds

1 teaspoon Dijon mustard

2 tablespoons nutritional yeast

¼ cup white wine vinegar

¼ teaspoon dried thyme (or ½ teaspoon chopped fresh thyme)

Preheat oven to 350 degrees F. Roast unpeeled garlic bulb in a small baking dish for about 25 minutes or until soft. When cool, squeeze out the soft cooked garlic, removing and discarding the skins.

Blend the garlic with the non-dairy milk, almonds, pumpkin seeds, mustard, nutritional yeast and vinegar in a high-powered blender until creamy and smooth. Stir in thyme.

CALORIES 173; PROTEIN 9g; CARBOHYDRATES 8g; SUGARS 1g; TOTAL FAT 12g; SATURATED FAT 1.2g; SODIUM 37mg; FIBER 3g

Cantaloupe or other fruit for dessert

> **Tip:** Select tomato products that use BPA-free packaging.

DINNER

CUBAN BLACK BEANS
4 SERVINGS

¾ cup chopped onion

¾ cup chopped green bell pepper

1 ⅓ cups no-salt-added or low-sodium tomato juice

3 cups cooked black beans, or 2 (15 ounce) cans, no-salt-added or low sodium, drained

1 cup chopped tomatoes

⅔ cup no-salt-added or low-sodium tomato sauce

2 cloves garlic, minced

1 teaspoon cumin

½ teaspoon garlic powder

¼ teaspoon black pepper

Heat 2 tablespoons water in a large pot and water sauté the onion and pepper until tender. Add tomato juice and next 7 ingredients; bring to a boil. Cover, reduce heat, and simmer 20 to 25 minutes or until vegetables are tender.

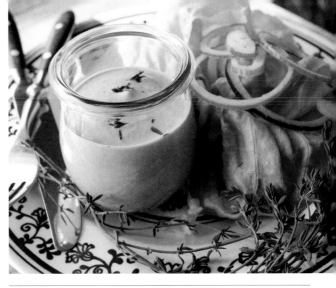

CALORIES 227; PROTEIN 14g; CARBOHYDRATES 43g; SUGARS 7g; TOTAL FAT 1g; SATURATED FAT 0.2g; SODIUM 82mg; FIBER 14g

Men: Have 2 servings of Cuban Black Beans.

Serve with 1 cup cooked quinoa per serving

Portion leftover Cuban Black Beans into individual containers. Use the remaining servings for alternate lunches or dinners over the next 3 to 4 days or freeze for later use.

FIVE MINUTE CHOCOLATE ICE CREAM
2 SERVINGS

2 tablespoons unsweetened soy, hemp or almond milk

2 regular dates or 1 Medjool date

4 walnut halves

1-2 tablespoons unsweetened cocoa powder

1 teaspoon alcohol-free vanilla extract

2 large bananas, frozen (see note)

Add non-dairy milk, dates, walnuts, cocoa powder and vanilla to a high-powered blender and start to blend. Drop frozen banana pieces in slowly. Add additional non-dairy milk if needed to reach desired consistency.

Note: Freeze ripe bananas at least 8 hours in advance. Peel bananas and seal in a plastic bag before freezing.

CALORIES 223; PROTEIN 4g; CARBOHYDRATES 44g; SUGARS 26g; TOTAL FAT 6g; SATURATED FAT 0.8g; SODIUM 10mg; FIBER 6g

Freeze the leftover serving of ice cream and enjoy it over the next few days, whenever you need a dessert treat.

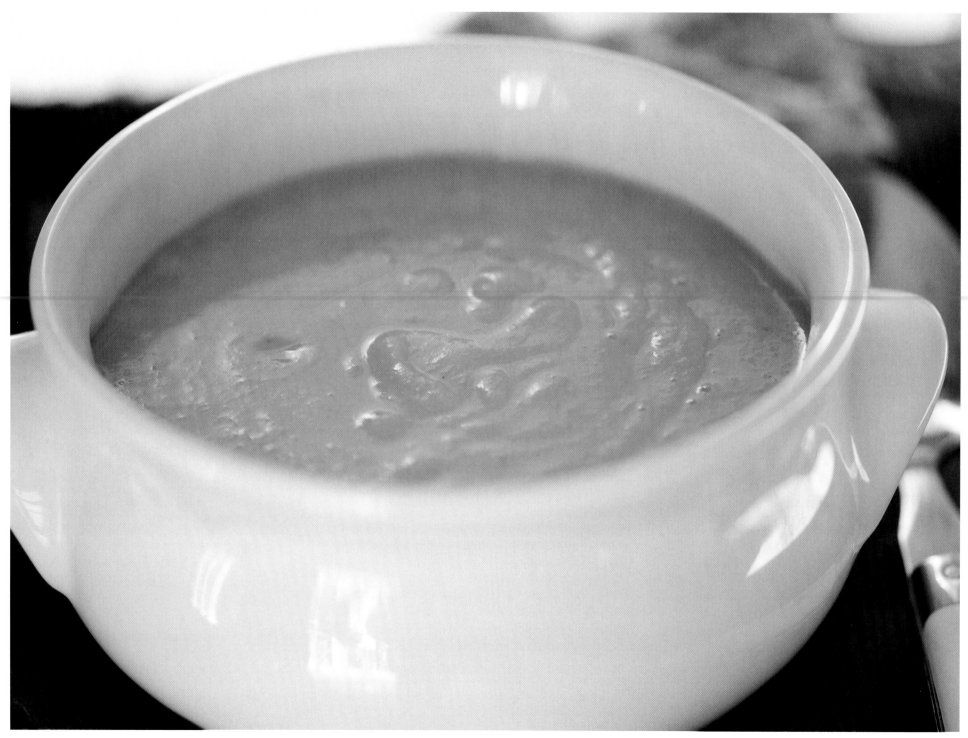

DAY 5

It takes time for your taste buds to adapt to this new way of eating. Be patient with yourself while you adapt to the lower levels of salt, sugar and oil in natural foods. Over time, you will find that you enjoy this style of eating every bit as much, and even more than your prior diet.

BREAKFAST

TOFU SCRAMBLE WITH TOMATOES AND PEPPERS
1 SERVING

½ cup chopped green or red pepper

¼ cup chopped onion

1 clove garlic, chopped

1 cup chopped tomatoes

7 ounces extra-firm tofu, drained and crumbled

1 cup firmly-packed spinach

½ teaspoon garlic powder

¼ teaspoon turmeric

¼ teaspoon red pepper flakes or ⅛ teaspoon chipotle chili powder (or to taste)

Heat 2-3 tablespoons water in a large skillet and water sauté peppers, onion and garlic until tender. Add remaining ingredients and cook for another five minutes.

CALORIES 258; PROTEIN 22g; CARBOHYDRATES 23g; SUGARS 9g; TOTAL FAT 10g; SATURATED FAT 1.3g; SODIUM 90mg; FIBER 7g

Fresh or thawed frozen strawberries

LUNCH

KALE SALAD WITH AVOCADO AND APPLES

(or leftover Chickpea Tuno Salad from Day 3 lunch with romaine lettuce and tomatoes)
1 SERVING

5 cups chopped kale

⅓ avocado, peeled and chopped

1 tablespoon lemon juice

1 apple, cored and chopped

½ cup cooked (or canned) cannellini beans or other beans

1 clove garlic, minced

½ teaspoon fresh ginger root, minced

2 tablespoons minced onion

Roll up each kale leaf and slice thinly. Add to bowl along with avocado and lemon juice. Using your hands, massage lemon juice and avocado into kale leaves until kale starts to soften and wilt and each leaf is coated, about 2 to 3 minutes. Mix in apple, beans, garlic, ginger and onion.

CALORIES 386; PROTEIN 21g; CARBOHYDRATES 81g; SUGARS 8g; TOTAL FAT 3g; SATURATED FAT 0.5g; SODIUM 152mg; FIBER 17g

Men: Add a half cup of cooked quinoa or farro to the salad or have the rest of the avocado.

DINNER

QUICK CREAMY CAULIFLOWER SOUP
4 SERVINGS

1 medium onion, chopped

2 cloves garlic

1 head cauliflower, chopped

2 cups carrot juice

4-5 cups low-sodium or no-salt-added vegetable broth

¼ cup raw cashews

¼ cup hemp seeds

1 teaspoon no-salt seasoning blend such as Dr. Fuhrman's VegiZest or Mrs. Dash, adjusted to taste

¼ teaspoon curry powder

¼ teaspoon ground turmeric

¼ cup chopped fresh dill

Heat 2-3 tablespoons of water in a soup pot, add onion and garlic and sauté until soft. Add cauliflower, carrot juice and 4 cups of the vegetable broth, bring to a boil, reduce heat and simmer for 25 minutes or until cauliflower is very tender. Working in batches, blend soup with hemp seeds and cashews in a high-powered blender.

Return to soup pot and reheat before serving. Season with no-salt seasoning, curry powder and turmeric. Stir in dill. If desired, add additional vegetable broth to adjust consistency.

CALORIES 218; PROTEIN 9g; CARBOHYDRATES 28g; SUGARS 9g; TOTAL FAT 9g; SATURATED FAT 1.3g; SODIUM 262mg; FIBER 6g

Portion leftover Quick Creamy Cauliflower Soup into individual containers. If you are busy tomorrow, have it for lunch and use the remaining servings over the next 3 to 4 days or freeze for later use.

Tip: Soups and stews are critical components of this eating style. When vegetables are simmered in broth, all the nutrients remain there.

ONION AND GARLIC-BRAISED GREENS
2 SERVINGS

1 small onion, thinly sliced

2 cloves garlic, thinly sliced

10 ounces chopped kale, collards or other greens (see tip)

¼ cup low-sodium or no-salt-added vegetable broth

⅛ teaspoon red pepper flakes, or to taste

1 teaspoon white wine vinegar, or to taste

Heat 2-3 tablespoons water in a large wok or sauté pan. Add onion and garlic and water sauté until onion is tender, about 3 minutes. Gradually add greens, and cook until wilted. Add broth and red pepper flakes, cover and cook over low-medium heat until greens are tender, about 6-8 minutes. Add more broth or water, if needed, to prevent sticking. Stir in vinegar.

CALORIES 92; PROTEIN 5g; CARBOHYDRATES 19g; SUGARS 1g; TOTAL FAT 1g; SATURATED FAT 0.1g; SODIUM 80mg; FIBER 4g

Tip: To save time, look for bags of prewashed, pre-chopped kale or collards.

DAYS 6-10
SHOPPING LIST

This shopping list assumes that all recipes in the meal plan will be made. Menus frequently include fruit for dessert and will mention a specific fruit as an example. That fruit is used for the shopping list.

Check your refrigerator, freezer and pantry before shopping. You may have items leftover from Days 1-5 that you can use. Make sure you also have all the items listed in the Stock Your Pantry list.

FRESH PRODUCE

VEGETABLES

- [ ] 15 ounces mixed salad greens (about 15 cups)
- [ ] 2 heads romaine lettuce
- [ ] 3 ounces baby kale (about 2 cups; increase to 4 cups for men)
- [ ] 5 ounces spinach (about 5 cups)
- [ ] Watercress (need 3 cups)
- [ ] Arugula (need 1 cup)
- [ ] 1 large head broccoli
- [ ] Your choice of a 2 green vegetables to equal 2 cups cooked for each (could also buy frozen)
- [ ] 5 green bell peppers (3 should be large enough to stuff)
- [ ] ¾ pound Brussels sprouts
- [ ] 1 zucchini
- [ ] 2 medium-large eggplants
- [ ] 1 butternut squash (need 2 cups chopped)
- [ ] 1 leek
- [ ] 2 Portobello mushrooms
- [ ] 8 ounces white or cremini mushrooms
- [ ] 5 medium tomatoes
- [ ] 3 avocados

- [ ] 1 carrot
- [ ] 2 bulbs garlic
- [ ] 3 shallots
- [ ] 5 yellow onions
- [ ] 1 red onion
- [ ] Parsley (any left from Days 1-5?)
- [ ] Cilantro
- [ ] Basil
- [ ] Fresh thyme (could use dry thyme)
- [ ] Fresh rosemary (could use dry rosemary)

FRUIT

- [ ] 2 ½ cups (3 cups for men) blueberries (could also use frozen)
- [ ] 2 cups fresh strawberries
- [ ] 1 honeydew melon
- [ ] 3 apples
- [ ] 2 navel oranges
- [ ] 2 kiwi
- [ ] 1 banana
- [ ] 2 lemons
- [ ] 1 lime

REFRIGERATED

- [ ] 2 cups (2 ½ for men) unsweetened, unflavored soy, hemp or almond milk
- [ ] 6 ounces lean ground turkey, optional

FROZEN

This list does not include vegetables and fruit listed under fresh produce that have a frozen option.

- [ ] Peaches (need 8 ounces)
- [ ] Corn (need ½ cup)

SHELF STABLE

BEANS

It is assumed that canned low-sodium or no-salt-added beans will be used. If you opt to start with dry beans, 1 cup of dry beans will yield about 3 cups of cooked beans.

- [ ] 4 (15 ounce) cans kidney or pinto beans
- [ ] 3 (15 ounce) cans black beans
- [ ] 2 (15 ounce) cans cannellini or other white beans

NUTS

- [ ] ¼ cup pecans

OTHER

Choose tomato products packaged in BPA-free materials.

- [ ] 3 (32 ounce) cartons no-salt-added or low-sodium vegetable broth (need about 10 cups)
- [ ] Low-sodium tomato sauce (need 1 ½ cups)
- [ ] Tomato paste (need 2 tablespoons)
- [ ] No-salt-added diced tomatoes (need 1 ½ cups)
- [ ] Dried porcini mushrooms (need ½ cup)
- [ ] Low-sodium ketchup (need 3 tablespoons)

DAY 6

The number of people with type 2 diabetes is rapidly increasing, having tripled in America over the last 30 years. The main reason for this is openly recognized: America's rapidly expanding waistline. The explosion in the occurrence of diabetes in the last 30 years in America parallels the skyrocketing number of overweight people.

BREAKFAST

BLUEBERRY NUT STEEL-CUT OATS
1 SERVING

1 cup water
¼ cup steel-cut oats (see note and tip)
½ cup diced apple
1 tablespoon ground flax seeds
½ cup fresh or frozen blueberries
1 tablespoon chopped walnuts or pecans

In a saucepan, bring water to a boil and stir in all ingredients, except blueberries and nuts. Reduce heat, cover, and simmer for 15 minutes or until oats are tender and water is absorbed, stirring occasionally. Stir in blueberries and nuts and heat for another minute.

Note: To make with old-fashioned rolled oats instead of steel cut, use ½ cup oats and reduce cooking time to 5 minutes.

CALORIES 377; PROTEIN 11g; CARBOHYDRATES 52g; SUGARS 14 g; TOTAL FAT 16g; SATURATED FAT 1.2g; SODIUM 13mg; FIBER 11g

Tip: Steel-cut oats are oat kernels that have been chopped into thick pieces. Since they are an intact whole grain they are digested more slowly than old-fashioned rolled oats which have been steamed and rolled into thin flakes. Steel-cut oats cause less of a spike in blood sugar and are a good choice, particularly for those with diabetes.

LUNCH

Baba Ganoush served with tomato wedges on a bed of mixed greens (or leftover Quick Creamy Cauliflower Soup from Day 5 dinner served with raw vegetables dipped in leftover Creamy Roasted Garlic Dressing from Day 4 lunch)

QUICK BABA GANOUSH
2 SERVINGS

1 (1 ½ pound) eggplant
1 clove garlic, chopped
2 tablespoons fresh lemon Juice
2 tablespoons unhulled sesame seeds or tahini
2 tablespoons chopped flat leaf parsley

Preheat oven to 350 degrees F. Prick eggplant with a fork and place on a lightly oiled baking sheet.

Bake for 50 minutes or until soft, turning occasionally. Let cool and peel. Place eggplant and remaining ingredients in a food processor and puree until smooth.

CALORIES 140; PROTEIN 5g; CARBOHYDRATES 23g; SUGARS 4 g; TOTAL FAT 5g; SATURATED FAT 0.7g; SODIUM 10mg; FIBER 13g

2 kiwis or other fruit for dessert

Men: Add a serving of a leftover soup or 1 cup cooked quinoa or farro

DINNER

SUNNY BEAN BURGERS
6 BURGERS

3 cups cooked kidney or pinto beans or 2 (15 ounce) cans no-salt-added or low-sodium beans, drained
⅓ cup sunflower seeds, chopped
½ cup minced onion
3 tablespoons low-sodium ketchup
2 tablespoons old-fashioned rolled oats or more if needed
1 teaspoon chili powder

Preheat the oven to 350 degrees F. Mash the beans with a fork (or pulse in a food processor) and combine with the remaining ingredients. Form into six patties.

Place the patties on a lightly oiled or parchment paper lined baking sheet. Bake for 25 minutes. Remove from the oven and let cool slightly, until you can pick up each patty and compress it firmly in

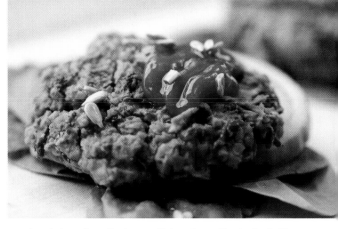

your hands to re-form the burger. Return the patties to the baking sheet, bottom side up, and bake for another 10 minutes.

CALORIES 178; PROTEIN 10g; CARBOHYDRATES 26g; SUGARS 3g; TOTAL FAT 5g; SATURATED FAT 0.5g; SODIUM 12mg; FIBER 8g

Serve with lettuce, sliced tomato and sliced red onion on a 100 percent whole grain pita (cut open to make 2 flat pieces) or on a bed of greens. (If using a pita, have one burger; have two if serving on greens.)

Wrap leftover burgers individually and freeze. They work well as a quick lunch or dinner.

SHREDDED BRUSSELS SPROUTS
2 SERVINGS

2 cloves garlic, chopped
¾ pound Brussels sprouts, cut into ⅛ inch ribbons
¼ cup toasted walnuts, chopped (see note)
2 tablespoons raisins
1 tablespoon nutritional yeast
freshly ground black pepper

Heat 2 tablespoons water in a large skillet and sauté garlic for 1 minute, add shredded Brussels sprouts and cook for 2-3 minutes, until warm and slightly wilted. Add a small amount of additional water if needed to prevent from sticking.

Remove from heat and toss with chopped, toasted walnuts, raisins and nutritional yeast. Season with black pepper.

Note: Toast walnuts in a small skillet over medium heat for 2-3 minutes or until lightly toasted.

CALORIES 200; PROTEIN 10g; CARBOHYDRATES 26g; SUGARS 10g; TOTAL FAT 9g; SATURATED FAT 0.9g; SODIUM 45mg; FIBER 9g

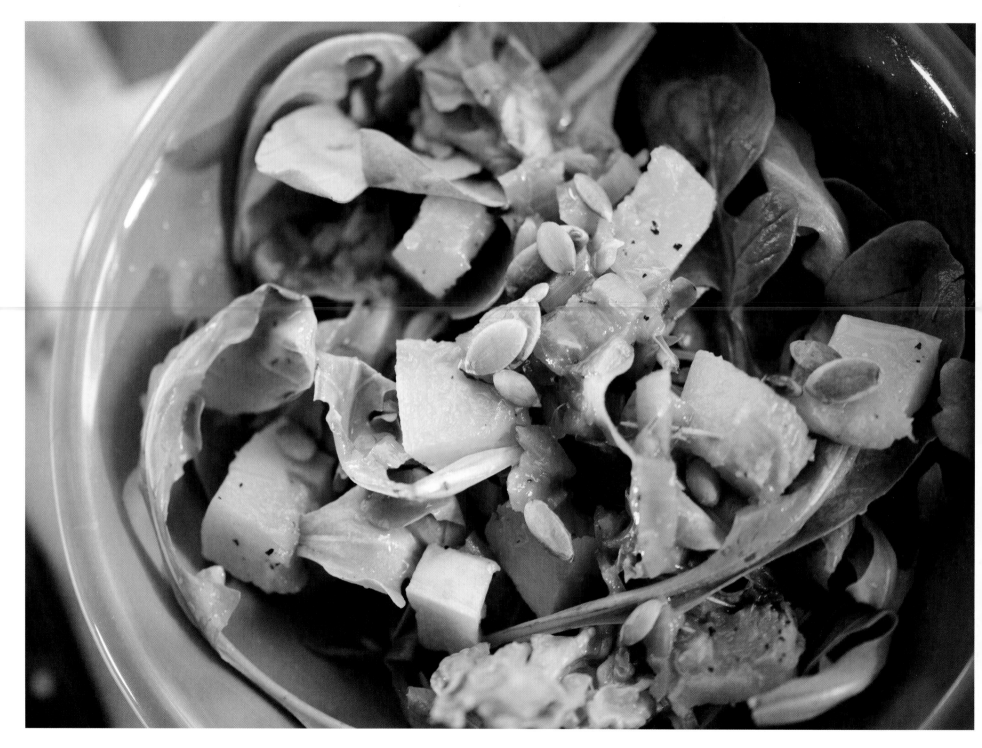

DAY 7

Natural plants, like vegetables and beans, contain thousands of protective micronutrients, such as antioxidants and phytochemicals. When we eat a diet rich in colorful plant foods, we obtain a full symphony of nutritional factors that our bodies need for optimal cell function and resistance to aging and stress.

BREAKFAST
SUPER EASY BLENDED SALAD
1 SERVING

8 ounces mixed salad greens
1 navel orange, peeled and seeded
juice of ¼ lemon

Blend ingredients in a high-powered blender until smooth and creamy.

CALORIES 119; PROTEIN 6g; CARBOHYDRATES 26g; SUGARS 15g; TOTAL FAT 1g; SATURATED FAT 0.2g; SODIUM 57mg; FIBER 8g

LUNCH
BUTTERNUT SQUASH SALAD WITH TOASTED PUMPKIN SEEDS
1 SERVING

2 cups butternut squash, peeled and cubed
¼ teaspoon black pepper, divided
2 medium shallots, minced
¼ cup balsamic vinegar
2 tablespoons water
2 teaspoons Dijon mustard
5 cups mixed salad greens
2 tablespoons raw pumpkin seeds, lightly toasted (see note)

Preheat oven to 350 degrees F. Arrange squash in a single layer on a lightly oiled or parchment paper lined baking pan. Sprinkle with ¼ teaspoon black pepper. Bake for 35 minutes or until squash is tender and lightly browned, stirring every fifteen minutes. Remove from oven, keep warm.

Water sauté shallots until tender. In a small bowl, whisk together shallots, balsamic vinegar, water and Dijon mustard. Place salad greens in a large bowl. Drizzle desired amount of vinegar mixture over greens and toss gently to coat. Top with warm butternut squash and pumpkin seeds.

Note: Toast pumpkin seeds in oven at 300 degrees F for 4 minutes, or until lightly toasted, stirring occasionally.

CALORIES 328; PROTEIN 12g; CARBOHYDRATES 55g; SUGARS 20g; TOTAL FAT 9g; SATURATED FAT 1.6g; SODIUM 173mg; FIBER 11g

Blueberries or other fruit for dessert.

DINNER
BLACK BEAN QUINOA SOUP
4 SERVINGS

1 medium onion, chopped
1 green bell pepper, chopped
4 cloves garlic, minced
1 cup chopped fresh tomato
1 teaspoon ground cumin
2 teaspoons chili powder
¼ teaspoon crushed red pepper flakes
1 large carrot, chopped
5 cups low-sodium or no-salt-added vegetable broth
½ cup dry quinoa, rinsed
3 cups cooked black beans or 2 (15 ounce) cans low-sodium or no-salt-added black beans, drained
4 cups packed baby spinach
¼ cup chopped cilantro
1 tablespoon fresh lime juice

In a soup pot, heat 2-3 tablespoons water, add onion and green pepper and water sauté until tender, about 5 minutes. Add more water, if needed, to prevent sticking. Add garlic and sauté another 30 seconds, until fragrant.

Add the tomatoes, cumin, chili powder and red pepper flakes and cook for 2-3 minutes, until tomatoes soften. Add carrots and vegetable broth, bring to a boil. Stir in the quinoa, reduce heat, cover and cook for 10 minutes. Add black beans and continue cooking until heated through and quinoa is tender, about 10 minutes. Add spinach and stir until wilted.

Remove from heat and stir in cilantro and lime juice.

CALORIES 317; PROTEIN 17g; CARBOHYDRATES 58g; SUGARS 4g; TOTAL FAT 3g; SATURATED FAT 0.4g; SODIUM 237mg; FIBER 16g

Men: Add raw vegetables with leftover Baba Ganoush from Day 6 dinner.

PEACH SORBET
2 SERVINGS

8 ounces frozen peaches
2 tablespoons unsweetened soy, hemp or almond milk, or more as needed
2 regular dates or 1 Medjool date, pitted

Blend ingredients until smooth in a food processor or high-powered blender. Add additional non-dairy milk, if needed, to adjust consistency.

CALORIES 72; PROTEIN 2g; CARBOHYDRATES 17g; SUGARS 15 g; TOTAL FAT 1g; SATURATED FAT 0g; SODIUM 8mg; FIBER 2g

Freeze the other serving of sorbet and have it with lunch or dinner tomorrow.

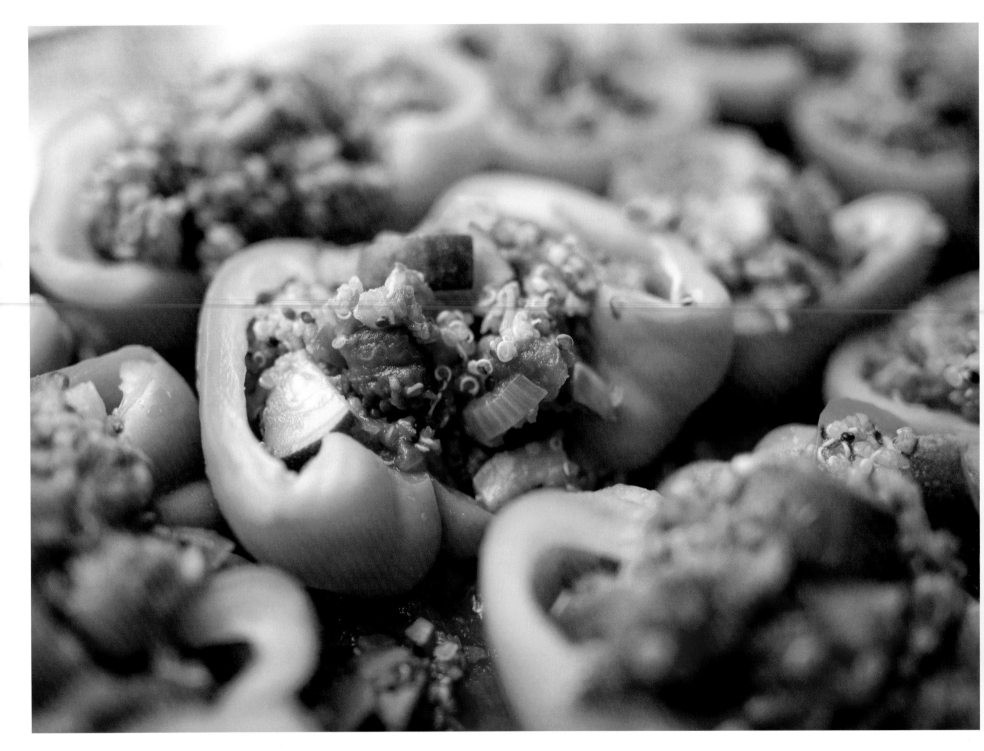

DAY 8

Green vegetables are so incredibly low in calories and rich in nutrients and fiber that the more of them you eat, the more weight you will lose.

BREAKFAST

BUCKWHEAT AND BERRIES CEREAL
1 SERVING

¼ cup raw buckwheat groats, rinsed (see note)
½ cup unsweetened soy, hemp or almond milk
¼ teaspoon cinnamon
¼ teaspoon alcohol-free vanilla extract
1 apple, chopped or grated
½ tablespoon raw almond or cashew butter
1 tablespoon chia seeds
½ cup fresh or thawed frozen blueberries or other berries

Place buckwheat, non-dairy milk, cinnamon and vanilla in a pan. Bring to a boil, reduce heat, cover and simmer for 6 minutes or until groats are soft, but not mushy, and almost all liquid is absorbed. Stir in apple, nut butter and chia seeds and simmer for another minute.

Stir in berries. Add additional non-dairy milk, if desired. May be refrigerated and eaten cold or reheated.

Note: Buckwheat groats are seeds from the buckwheat plant. They are unrelated to wheat and do not contain gluten. Choose raw buckwheat groats, not kasha, which is toasted.

CALORIES 369; PROTEIN 10g; CARBOHYDRATES 65g; SUGARS 21g; TOTAL FAT 10g; SATURATED FAT 1.0g; SODIUM 101mg; FIBER 12g

LUNCH

Big Green Salad with Avocado Dressing, include romaine lettuce, watercress, tomatoes, red onions, cannellini or other beans and pumpkin seeds (or Black Bean Quinoa Soup from Day 7 dinner and a sliced tomato, avocado and red onion salad)

AVOCADO DRESSING
2 SERVINGS

1 ripe avocado, peeled, pitted and chopped
1 tablespoon nutritional yeast
2 tablespoons unsweetened soy, hemp or almond milk
1 small shallot
2 tablespoons white wine vinegar

Blend all ingredients in a high-powered blender until smooth and creamy.

CALORIES 143; PROTEIN 4g; CARBOHYDRATES 9g; SUGARS 1g; TOTAL FAT 11g; SATURATED FAT 1.5g; SODIUM 14mg; FIBER 6g

Tip: Unlike most fruits, avocados start to ripen only after they are picked. Unripe, firm and green fruit can take four to five days to ripen. A ripe avocado yields to gentle pressure but is still firm. If your avocado is ripe before you are ready to eat it, it can be refrigerated to slow down the ripening process.

DINNER

STUFFED PEPPERS WITH QUINOA, EGGPLANT AND BASIL (with optional ground turkey)
3 SERVINGS

½ cup dry quinoa, rinsed
3 large bell peppers, cut in half lengthwise, seeds and membranes removed
3 cloves garlic, minced
1 onion, minced
6 ounces lean ground turkey, optional
1 medium eggplant, diced
1 medium zucchini, diced
8 ounces mushrooms, diced
1 ½ cups low-sodium or no-salt-added tomato sauce or no-salt-added crushed or diced tomatoes
1 teaspoon Dr. Fuhrman's MatoZest, Italian seasoning or oregano (or to taste)
2 tablespoons fresh basil

In a saucepan, bring 1 cup water to a boil. Add quinoa, turn down the heat to low, cover and simmer gently until all the liquid is absorbed, about 15 minutes. Set aside.

Steam bell peppers, cut side down over ½ inch boiling water until nearly tender, about 8-10 minutes.

Heat ⅛ cup water and sauté the garlic and onion. If using ground turkey, add and continue to sauté until meat is cooked through. Add the eggplant, zucchini and mushrooms and cook until eggplant and zucchini are soft. Stir in the cooked quinoa, tomato sauce or crushed tomatoes, seasonings and basil. Spoon vegetable/quinoa mixture into peppers.

Serve immediately or if desired, bake for 15 minutes at 350 degrees F.

CALORIES 255; PROTEIN 12g; CARBOHYDRATES 49g; SUGARS 17g; TOTAL FAT 3g; SATURATED FAT 0.4g; SODIUM 27mg; FIBER 14g

Orange or other fruit for dessert (or leftover peach sorbet from day 7 dinner)

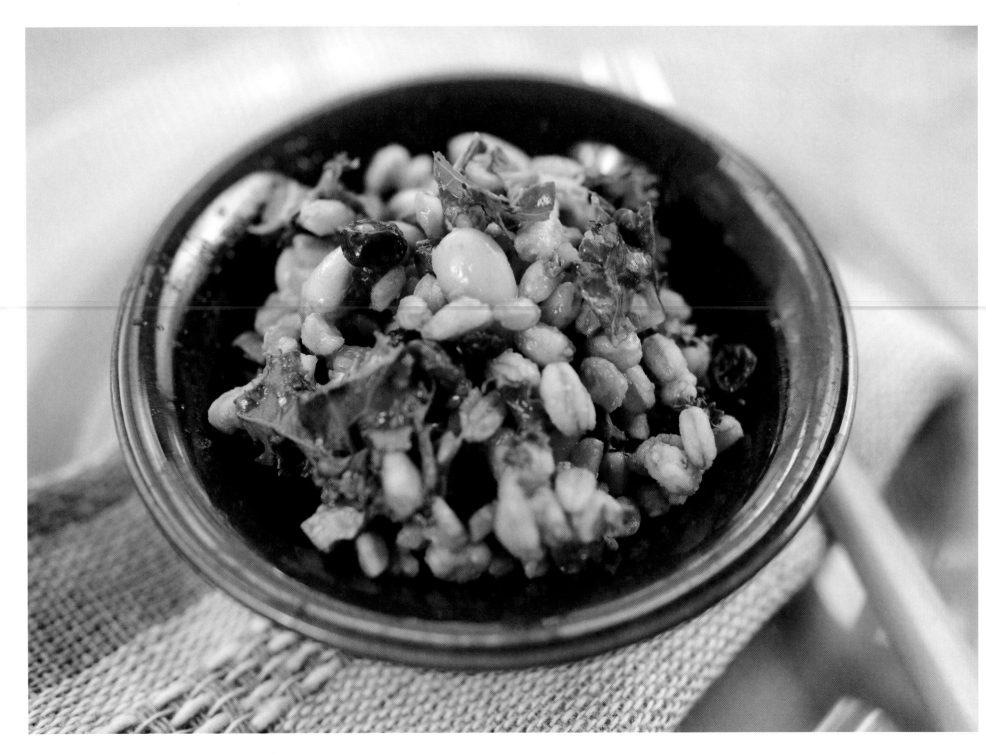

DAY 9

The fiber and resistant starch in beans powerfully reduces hunger. Eating beans will reduce your appetite for many hours, overall lowering the amount of calories you desire for the day.

BREAKFAST

BREAKFAST BROCCOLI
2 SERVINGS

1 large head broccoli florets and stems
1 avocado, peeled, pitted and diced
1 leek
black pepper, to taste
1 tablespoon sesame seeds

Steam broccoli (florets and stems) and the leek in a steamer, until everything is soft enough to blend. Process broccoli, leek and diced avocado in a blender or food processor until a creamy consistency is reached. Season with black pepper and sprinkle with sesame seeds.

If desired, place in a baking dish and bake for 12 minutes on top rack at 350 degrees F.

CALORIES 270; PROTEIN 11g; CARBOHYDRATES 34g; SUGARS 7g; TOTAL FAT 14g; SATURATED FAT 1.9g; SODIUM 115mg; FIBER 14g

Honeydew melon or other fruit
Men: Replace fruit with Eat Your Beans Green Smoothie from Day 3.

LUNCH

FARRO AND KALE SALAD WITH WHITE BEANS AND WALNUTS
2 SERVINGS

½ cup farro
1 ½ cups low-sodium or no-salt-added vegetable broth plus an additional ¼ cup for the dressing
2 cups whole baby kale leaves or chopped kale
½ cup cooked cannellini or other white beans
2 tablespoons raisins
2 tablespoons walnut pieces (or lightly toasted pine nuts)
1 teaspoon chia seeds
2 tablespoons balsamic vinegar
1 tablespoon fresh lemon juice
1 teaspoon Dijon mustard
ground black pepper, to taste

Place farro in a pot with 1 ½ cups of the vegetable broth, and bring to a boil. Reduce heat to a simmer. Cover the pot and cook for 25 to 40 minutes, until grains are tender, but not split, and have absorbed all of the liquid (or cook according to package instructions). Remove from heat and transfer to a large bowl.

To the farro, add the kale, white beans, raisins and walnuts. Stir to allow the warm farro to wilt the kale.

To make the dressing, whisk together the chia seeds, the remaining ¼ cup of the vegetable broth, vinegar, lemon juice, mustard and pepper in a small bowl. Allow to stand for 15 minutes to thicken.

Toss farro salad with enough dressing to moisten it, but not make it too wet.

CALORIES 385; PROTEIN 14g; CARBOHYDRATES 71g; SUGARS 9g; TOTAL FAT 7g; SATURATED FAT 0.7g; SODIUM 207mg; FIBER 14g

DINNER

PORTOBELLO STEAKS WITH PECAN HERB GRAVY
1 SERVING

2 Portobello mushroom caps
1 tablespoon plus 1 teaspoon balsamic vinegar
1 clove garlic, minced
1 tablespoon minced fresh rosemary leaves (or 1 teaspoon dried rosemary)
1 tablespoon minced fresh thyme (or 1 teaspoon dried thyme)
1 tablespoon minced fresh parsley
1 cup diced onion
1 teaspoon Bragg Liquid Aminos
1 cup low-sodium or no-salt-added vegetable broth
¼ cup pecans, lightly toasted
2 teaspoons nutritional yeast
½ cup dried porcini mushrooms, soaked in ½ cup water for 30 minutes, drained (reserve soaking water) and then diced

Preheat oven to 350 degrees F. Place the Portobello caps, gill side facing up, on a baking sheet. In a small bowl, mix together one tablespoon of the balsamic vinegar, garlic, rosemary, thyme and parsley. Reserve half of this mixture to use for the gravy. Divide the remaining portion between the Portobello caps and rub onto each one. Bake for 30 minutes.

To make the gravy, heat a skillet over medium heat and sauté the remaining vinegar and herb mixture along with the diced onion, Bragg Liquid Aminos and 1 tablespoon of the vegetable broth. Cook and stir for 5 minutes or until the onion is tender.

Place the pecans in a high-powered blender and blend with ½ cup of the vegetable broth until smooth. Add this to the sautéed herbs and onion, along with the nutritional yeast, remaining broth, soaked dried porcini mushrooms and their soaking liquid. Bring to a gentle boil. Reduce heat to simmer on low for 5 to 10 minutes. Serve hot, over the baked Portobello caps.

CALORIES 236; PROTEIN 9g; CARBOHYDRATES 31g; SUGARS 11g; TOTAL FAT 11g; SATURATED FAT 1.1g; SODIUM 203mg; FIBER 7g

If you have extra pecan gravy, refrigerate it. You can use it with other cooked vegetables.

Your choice of a cooked, green vegetable (can use fresh or frozen)

Strawberries or other fruit for dessert

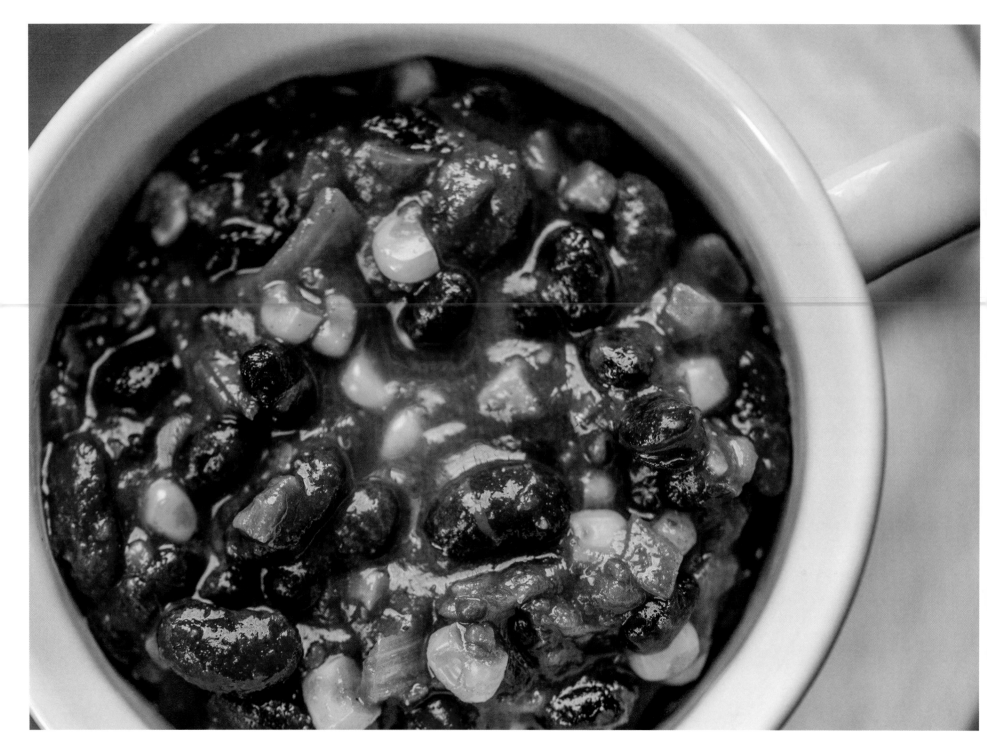

DAY 10

Beans and greens are the foods closely linked in the scientific literature with protection against cancer, diabetes, heart disease, stroke and dementia.

Tip: When choosing a whole-grain bread, pita or wrap, read the ingredient list to make sure it is 100 percent whole grain. It should list "whole" grain as the first ingredient and if more than one grain is used, they should all be whole grains.

BREAKFAST

Nutritarian Granola with non-dairy milk and ½ cup fresh or thawed frozen strawberries

NUTRITARIAN GRANOLA
5 SERVINGS

⅓ cup raw almond or cashew butter
1 apple, peeled, quartered
½ ripe banana
1 teaspoon ground cinnamon
¼ teaspoon ground nutmeg
1 teaspoon alcohol-free vanilla extract
2 cups old-fashioned rolled oats
½ cup chopped raw walnuts or pecans
¼ cup raw pumpkin seeds
2 tablespoons unsweetened shredded coconut

Preheat oven to 225 degrees F.

Place the nut butter, apple, banana, cinnamon, nutmeg and vanilla extract in a high-powered blender and blend until smooth

In a large bowl, mix the oats, nuts, seeds and coconut. Add the blended mixture and toss to combine. Transfer mixture to a parchment-lined baking pan. Do not overcrowd the pan so the granola can bake evenly. Bake for 30 minutes, stirring occasionally. Allow to cool, then store in an airtight container.

CALORIES 366; PROTEIN 10g; CARBOHYDRATES 36g; SUGARS 5g; TOTAL FAT 23g; SATURATED FAT 4.6g; SODIUM 4mg; FIBER 6g

Use the leftover granola as an alternate breakfast. Sprinkle some on a bowl of berries for a quick and easy option.

LUNCH

ARUGULA AND SPINACH STUFFED PITAS WITH WATERCRESS PESTO
PESTO: 3 SERVINGS; PITA: 1 SERVING

For the Pesto:
1 bulb garlic
2 cups watercress, stems removed
5 basil leaves
½ cup walnuts
¼ cup unsweetened soy, hemp or almond milk

For the Sandwich:
1 (100% whole grain) pita
½ tomato, sliced
¼ onion, thinly sliced
1 cup arugula
1 cup spinach
¼ avocado, sliced

Cut top ¼ inch off garlic bulb and lightly roast for 15 minutes at 300 degrees F. Cut open cloves and squeeze out soft cooked garlic. Blend the roasted garlic with the other pesto ingredients in a high-powered blender

Spread pesto on the whole grain pita and stuff with the remaining ingredients.

CALORIES 353; PROTEIN 12g; CARBOHYDRATES 39g; SUGARS 4g; TOTAL FAT 20g; SATURATED FAT 2.1g; SODIUM 175mg; FIBER 10g

Use leftover Watercress Pesto at dinner to season your cooked vegetable. You can add the leftover watercress, arugula and spinach to your salads.

Honeydew melon or other fruit for dessert

DINNER

TWO BEAN CHILI
4 SERVINGS

1 cup chopped onion
½ cup chopped green bell pepper
1 clove garlic, chopped
¾ cup water
2 tablespoons tomato paste
1 tablespoon chili powder
2 teaspoons ground cumin
¼ teaspoon black pepper
1 ½ cups cooked black beans or 1 (15 ounce) can low-sodium or no-salt-added black beans
3 cups cooked red pinto or kidney beans or 2 (15 ounce) cans low-sodium or no-salt-added red beans
1 ½ cups low-sodium or no-salt-added vegetable broth
1 ½ cups diced tomatoes
½ cup frozen corn kernels
1 tablespoon yellow cornmeal

Water sauté onion and bell pepper in a soup pot until almost tender. Add garlic and cook for another minute. Stir in water, tomato paste, chili powder, cumin, black pepper, beans, vegetable broth, diced tomatoes and corn and bring to a boil. Reduce heat, cover and simmer for 10 minutes. Stir in cornmeal and cook for an additional two minutes.

CALORIES 338; PROTEIN 20g; CARBOHYDRATES 64g; SUGARS 6g; TOTAL FAT 2g; SATURATED FAT 0.3g; SODIUM 120mg; FIBER 19g; BETA-CAROTENE 737ug; VITAMIN C 32mg; CALCIUM 107mg; IRON 7mg; FOLATE 299ug

Freeze a serving of the chili. It's on the menu again on Day 18.

Men: Have an extra serving of Two Bean Chili.

Your choice of a cooked green vegetable.

DAYS 11-15
SHOPPING LIST

This shopping list assumes that all recipes in the meal plan will be made. Menus frequently include fruit for dessert and will mention a specific fruit as an example. That fruit is used for the shopping list.

Check your refrigerator, freezer and pantry before shopping. You may have items leftover from Days 1-10 that you can use. Make sure you also have all the items listed in the Stock Your Pantry list.

FRESH PRODUCE

VEGETABLES

- [ ] 2 heads romaine lettuce
- [ ] 9 ounces kale (about 13 cups)
- [ ] 8 ounces spinach (about 8 cups)
- [ ] Collard greens (need 1 cup)
- [ ] Arugula (need 2 cups) any left from days 6-10?
- [ ] 1 green bell pepper
- [ ] 1 red bell pepper
- [ ] Raw vegetables of choice to eat with hummus
- [ ] 1 medium eggplant
- [ ] 1 medium butternut squash
- [ ] 2 sweet potatoes
- [ ] 28 ounces white or crimini mushrooms
- [ ] 5 medium tomatoes
- [ ] 1 avocado
- [ ] 8 carrots
- [ ] celery (need 9 stalks)
- [ ] 2 bulbs garlic
- [ ] 6 yellow onions
- [ ] 1 red onion
- [ ] Ginger (need 1 teaspoon chopped)
- [ ] Fresh mint
- [ ] Cilantro (any left from Days 6-10?)
- [ ] Basil (any left from Days 6-10?)

FRUIT

- [ ] 2 cups strawberries (could also use frozen)
- [ ] 2 cups (3 cups for men) blueberries (could also use frozen)
- [ ] 4 apples
- [ ] 1 ½ cups fresh pineapple (could also use frozen)
- [ ] 1 orange
- [ ] 2 lemons
- [ ] 1 lime
- [ ] Add 1 banana for men

REFRIGERATED

- [ ] 5 cups unflavored, unsweetened soy, hemp or almond milk
- [ ] 6 ounces extra-firm tofu

FROZEN

This list does not include include vegetables and fruit listed under fresh produce that have a frozen option.

- [ ] Corn (need 1 cup) any left from Days 6-10?
- [ ] Cherries (need ½ cup) could substitute frozen blueberries

SHELF STABLE

BEANS

It is assumed that canned, low-sodium or no-salt-added beans will be used. If you opt to start with dry beans, 1 cup of dry beans will yield about 3 cups of cooked beans

- [ ] 2 (15 ounce) cans pinto or black beans
- [ ] 1 (15 ounce) can (2 for men) chickpeas
- [ ] 1 (15 ounce) can cannellini or other white beans
- [ ] 1 (15 ounce) can (2 for men) any variety beans
- [ ] 1 pound dry split peas
- [ ] Dry lentils (need 1 cup)
- [ ] Edamame in the pod

OTHER

Choose tomato products packaged in in BPA-free materials.

- [ ] 3 (32 ounce) cartons no-salt-added or low-sodium vegetable broth (need about 12 cups)
- [ ] Low-sodium pasta sauce (need 1 ½ cups)
- [ ] Low-sodium tomato sauce (need 8 ounces)
- [ ] Tomato paste (need 1 tablespoon) any left from Days 6-10?
- [ ] Unsulfured, no-salt-added dried tomatoes (need 1 ounce)
- [ ] Low-sodium salsa (need 2 tablespoons)
- [ ] Hulled or hull-less (not pearled) barley (need 1 cup)
- [ ] 5 Corn tortillas (could substitute 100% whole grain flour tortillas)
- [ ] Dry sherry or sherry vinegar

DAY 11

This is not a fat-free eating style. Our bodies require healthy fats from whole foods. By eating healthy fats from nuts, seeds and avocados, we also receive the lignans, flavonoids, antioxidants, minerals and other protective phytochemicals that come along with the whole food package.

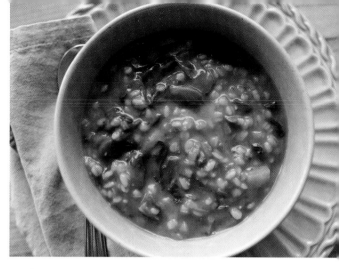

BREAKFAST

SAVORY STEEL-CUT OATS
2 SERVINGS

1 small onion, chopped

1 cup sliced mushrooms

1 cup steel-cut oats

2 cups no-salt-added or low-sodium vegetable broth

1 cup unsweetened soy, hemp or almond milk

2 tablespoons nutritional yeast

1 ½ teaspoons Cajun or other spicy, no-salt seasoning

1 ounce unsulfured, no-salt-added dried tomatoes, soaked until softened, chopped

3 cups spinach

Dry sauté onions in a non-stick pan for 1-2 minutes, then add mushrooms and continue to sauté until vegetables are tender.

Add onion and mushroom mixture and remaining ingredients except spinach to a pot, heat to boiling, reduce heat, and simmer, stirring occasionally, until the water is absorbed and the oats are creamy, about 20 minutes.

Stir in the spinach, remove from heat, cover and let sit until the spinach is soft.

CALORIES 296; PROTEIN 17g; CARBOHYDRATES 46g; SUGARS 3g; TOTAL FAT 6g; SATURATED FAT 1g; SODIUM 115mg; FIBER 10g

Fresh or thawed frozen blueberries

LUNCH

CAESAR'S SECRET SALAD
SALAD: 1 SERVING; DRESSING: 4 SERVINGS

For the Dressing:
6 cloves garlic

1 cup unsweetened soy, hemp or almond milk

1 cup raw cashews or ½ cup raw cashew butter

2 tablespoons nutritional yeast

2 tablespoons fresh lemon juice

1 tablespoon Dijon mustard

⅛ teaspoon black pepper

For the Salad:
1 head romaine lettuce, chopped or leaves left whole

2 tablespoons Nutritarian Parmesan (see note)

To make dressing, bake garlic cloves (leave papery skins on) at 350 degrees F for about 25 minutes or until garlic is soft. When cool, remove the skins. Blend roasted garlic and the remaining dressing ingredients in a high-powered blender. Toss romaine lettuce with Nutritarian Parmesan and desired amount of dressing.

Refrigerate leftover Caesar Dressing and use it for lunch tomorrow.

Note: To make Nutritarian Parmesan, place ¼ cup walnuts and ¼ cup nutritional yeast in a food processor and pulse until the texture of grated Parmesan is achieved. Store leftover in an airtight container and refrigerate. (Any leftover from Day 2 dinner?)

CALORIES 314; PROTEIN 17g; CARBOHYDRATES 22g; SUGARS 4g; TOTAL FAT 19g; SATURATED FAT 3.1g; SODIUM 85mg; FIBER 7g

Men: Add ½-1 cup beans (any variety) to the salad

Orange or other fruit for dessert

> **Tip:** If you are pressed for time and opt for a bottled dressing, use a no-oil dressing that contains no more than 75 mg of sodium per tablespoon. Add 1 to 2 tablespoons of raw nuts or seeds to the salad to enhance the absorption of nutrients.

DINNER

MUSHROOM AND BARLEY SOUP
4 SERVINGS

1 medium onion, chopped

1 cup chopped carrots

½ cup chopped celery

3 cloves garlic, minced

20 ounces mushrooms, sliced

1 teaspoon Bragg Liquid Aminos

1 cup hulled or hull-less barley (see note)

8 cups low-sodium or no-salt-added vegetable broth

¼ teaspoon ground black pepper or to taste

½ teaspoon dried thyme

2 cups arugula

Heat ¼ cup water in a large soup pot and water sauté onions, carrots, celery and garlic until softened, about 6 minutes. Add mushrooms and Bragg Liquid Aminos and cook until mushrooms release their juices, about 5 minutes. Add barley, vegetable broth, black pepper and thyme. Bring to a boil, reduce heat, cover and simmer for 60 minutes or until barley is tender. Stir in arugula and heat until it is wilted.

Note: Hulled barley and hull-less barley are two different varieties of barley; both are considered whole grains. Quicker cooking pearl barley has been refined and is not a whole grain.

CALORIES 255; PROTEIN 11g; CARBOHYDRATES 50g; SUGARS 6; TOTAL FAT 2g; SATURATED FAT 0.3g; SODIUM 106mg; FIBER 11g

Seasoned Edamame (Toss pods with a no-salt seasoning blend. Squeeze the beans out of the pods before eating.)

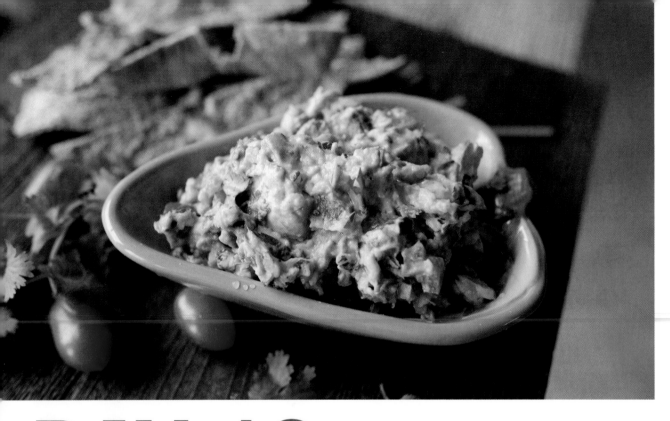

8 ounces no-salt-added or low-sodium tomato sauce, divided

2 cups cooked pinto or black beans or canned no-salt-added or low-sodium beans, drained

1 cup frozen corn kernels

1 tablespoon chili powder

1 teaspoon ground cumin

1 teaspoon onion powder

1 tablespoon chopped fresh cilantro

⅛ teaspoon cayenne pepper, or to taste

5 corn or (100% whole grain) flour tortillas

Sauté the green pepper and onion in 2 tablespoons of the tomato sauce until tender. Stir in the remaining tomato sauce, beans, corn, chili powder, cumin, onion powder, cilantro and cayenne. Simmer for 5 minutes.

Spoon about ¼ cup of the bean mixture on each tortilla and roll up. Serve as is or bake for 15 minutes in a 375 degree F oven.

CALORIES 290; PROTEIN 14g; CARBOHYDRATES 51g; SUGARS 1g; TOTAL FAT 4g; SATURATED FAT 0.7g; SODIUM 171mg; FIBER 13g

Men: Have 2 Bean Enchiladas.

Leftover beans can be used for tomorrow's Apple Bean Breakfast.

Tip: Spice it up if you like. A hint of spiciness from black pepper, cayenne pepper or red pepper flakes is sometimes just what a dish needs.

Raw Vegetables with Simple Guacamole

SIMPLE GUACAMOLE
2 SERVINGS

1 ripe avocado, peeled and pitted

¼ cup finely chopped onion

½ cup chopped tomato

1 small clove garlic, diced

2 tablespoons minced fresh cilantro

1 tablespoon fresh lime juice

⅛ teaspoon ground cumin

⅛ teaspoon freshly ground black pepper

Using a fork, mash the avocados in a small bowl. Add the remaining ingredients and stir well.

CALORIES 130; PROTEIN 2g; CARBOHYDRATES 10g; SUGARS 2g; TOTAL FAT 11g; SATURATED FAT 1.5g; SODIUM 8mg; FIBER 5g

DAY 12

Because nuts and seeds are rich in minerals and fiber and have a low glycemic index (GI), they are favorable foods to include in a diet designed for diabetics. They also reduce heart disease risk.

BREAKFAST

Nutritarian Granola (leftover from Day 10) with non-dairy milk and ½ cup fresh or thawed frozen strawberries

LUNCH

Big Salad with leftover Caesar Dressing (leftover from Day 11 lunch) (Salad should include romaine, arugula, tomatoes, red onions, and your choice of beans)

Apple or other fruit for dessert

DINNER

BEAN ENCHILADAS
5 SERVINGS

1 medium green bell pepper, seeded and chopped

½ cup sliced onion

DAY 13

Eat more foods rich in vegetable protein and less or no foods with animal protein. A diet high in animal products and low in vegetables and beans is the formula for a medical disaster. Diabetics need the opposite: a diet high in vegetables and beans and low in animal products.

BREAKFAST

APPLE BEAN BREAKFAST
1 SERVING

1 apple, cored and chopped
¼ cup water
1 teaspoon cinnamon
½ teaspoon nutmeg
1-2 cups chopped kale, spinach or collards
¼ cup cooked pinto, black or other beans
1 tablespoon raisins
2 tablespoons walnuts or other raw nuts

Place the chopped apple in a saucepan with the water. Begin cooking over medium-high heat. Add the remaining ingredients, stir, and cook until the apples are tender, about 5-10 minutes. Excess water can be drained off, if desired.

CALORIES 296; PROTEIN 8g; CARBOHYDRATES 48g; SUGARS 20g; TOTAL FAT 11g; SATURATED FAT 1.3g; SODIUM 36mg; FIBER 12g

Men: Increase beans to ½ cup and walnuts to ¼ cup.

LUNCH

BAKED TOFU PIZZA (or leftover Mushroom and Barley Soup from Day 11 dinner)
1 SERVING

6 ounces extra-firm tofu (about half a package)
½ cup low-sodium or no-salt-added pasta sauce
1 tablespoon tomato paste
½ teaspoon garlic powder

½ teaspoon onion powder

Cut tofu into thin slices and place on a wire rack.

Mix the spices with the tomato paste and tomato sauce and spread over the tofu. Bake in a 325 degree F oven for 30 minutes or until tofu is yellowed on the outside.

CALORIES 181; PROTEIN 15g; CARBOHYDRATES 19g; SUGARS 11g; TOTAL FAT 5g; SATURATED FAT 0.8g; SODIUM 157mg; FIBER 3g

---

Raw vegetables with Hummus (or leftover Guacamole from Day 12 dinner)

SUPER SIMPLE HUMMUS
4 SERVINGS

1 ½ cups cooked chickpeas or 1 (15 ounce) can no-salt-added or low-sodium chickpeas, drained
2 tablespoons lemon juice
2 tablespoons unhulled sesame seeds
1 clove garlic, minced
½ teaspoon ground cumin

Blend all ingredients in a high-powered blender or food processor. Add 1-2 tablespoons water if desired, to adjust consistency. Can be refrigerated for up to 4 days.

CALORIES 130; PROTEIN 6g; CARBOHYDRATES 19g; SUGARS 3g; TOTAL FAT 4g; SATURATED FAT 0.5g; SODIUM 5mg; FIBER 5g

---

DINNER

EASY SPLIT PEA STEW (or leftover Bean Enchiladas from Day 12 dinner)
3 SERVINGS

1 pound dry split peas, rinsed
7 cups low-sodium or no-salt-added vegetable broth
1 bay leaf
½ teaspoon dried thyme
1 teaspoon dried cumin
1 medium onion, chopped
4 stalks celery, thinly sliced
3 medium carrots, chopped
1 cup chopped mushrooms
2 cloves garlic, minced
4 cups packed spinach

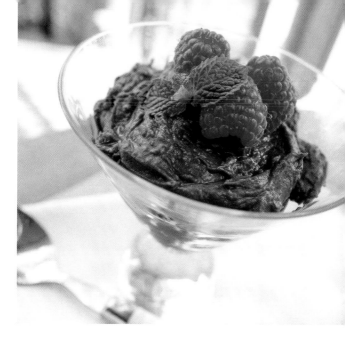

1 tablespoon dry sherry or sherry vinegar

In a large soup pot, combine split peas, broth, bay leaf, thyme and cumin. Bring to a boil, reduce heat, cover and simmer, for 45 minutes, stirring occasionally.

Stir in onion, celery, carrots, mushrooms and garlic. Return to a boil, reduce heat, cover, and simmer for an additional 20 to 25 minutes or until vegetables are tender. Stir in spinach and cook until wilted. Discard bay leaf. Stir in sherry.

CALORIES 348; PROTEIN 24g; CARBOHYDRATES 63g; SUGARS 10g; TOTAL FAT 1g; SATURATED FAT 0.2g; SODIUM 82mg; FIBER 25g

---

CHOCOLATE MOUSSE (top with fresh berries)
2 SERVINGS

2 medium sweet potatoes
½ cup frozen cherries or blueberries, thawed
4 tablespoons natural cocoa powder
¼ cup raw cashews
½ teaspoon alcohol-free vanilla or almond extract

Place sweet potatoes on a baking sheet and bake in a 350 degree F oven for 1 to 1 ½ hours until very tender. Remove skins. Place sweet potatoes, cherries, cocoa powder and vanilla in a high-powered blender and process until smooth and creamy.

CALORIES 249; PROTEIN 7g; CARBOHYDRATES 42g; SUGARS 10g; TOTAL FAT 9g; SATURATED FAT 2.2g; SODIUM 77mg; FIBER 10g

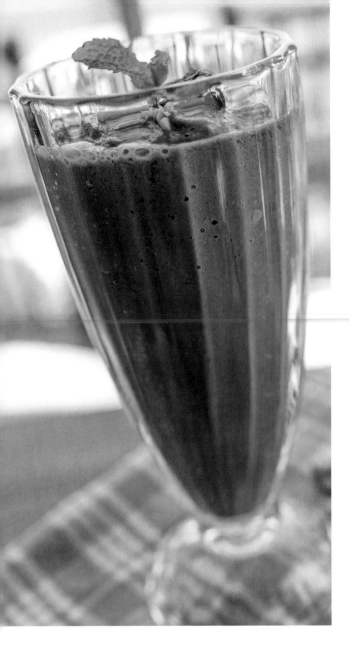

DAY 14

Medication is an insufficient and ineffective intervention for the chronic diseases that have been created by bad lifestyle and dietary choices.

BREAKFAST

WALDORF BLENDED SALAD
1 SERVING

⅓ cup unsweetened soy, hemp or almond milk

1 apple, peeled and cored

3 tablespoons chopped walnuts

2 cups kale and/or romaine lettuce

½ cup water or ice cubes

¼ teaspoon cinnamon

Blend all ingredients in high-powered blender.

CALORIES 269; PROTEIN 8g; CARBOHYDRATES 34g; SUGARS 14; TOTAL FAT 14g; SATURATED FAT 1.4g; SODIUM 125mg; FIBER 6g

Men: Add a Berry Bowl (Day 2 breakfast) or Chickpea Cereal (Day 16 breakfast).

LUNCH

LENTIL QUINOA SALAD
4 SERVINGS

1 cup dried lentils, rinsed

3 cups water

½ teaspoon dried thyme

1 garlic clove, chopped

¼ cup quinoa, rinsed

1 lemon, juiced

3 tablespoons balsamic or fruity-flavored vinegar

1 small onion, roughly chopped, divided

¼ cup raw cashews

2 tablespoons fresh mint leaves

1 teaspoon no-salt seasoning blend such as Dr. Fuhrman's VegiZest or Mrs. Dash (adjust to taste)

1 medium red bell pepper, chopped

1 orange, peeled and chopped

3 ounces (about 5 cups) kale, collards or other greens, tough stems removed, chopped (see note)

In a large saucepan, bring lentils and water to a boil with thyme and garlic. Reduce heat, cover and cook for 20 minutes, add the quinoa and cook for an additional 15 minutes or until lentils are tender.

Blend together lemon juice, vinegar, half of the onion, cashews, and mint leaves. Combine lentil mixture, remaining chopped onion, no-salt seasoning, pepper, orange and chopped greens and mix in desired amount of dressing. Chill before serving.

Note: The greens can be chopped up and mixed in with the salad or if desired, drop approximately 1/4 cup of the salad on top of whole collard, Swiss chard or romaine leaves and roll up.

CALORIES 348; PROTEIN 20g; CARBOHYDRATES 59g; SUGARS 8g; TOTAL FAT 6g; SATURATED FAT 1g; SODIUM 53mg; FIBER 20g

DINNER

EGGPLANT STACKS
2 SERVINGS

½ cup low-sodium or no-salt-added pasta sauce

1 medium eggplant, peeled and cut crosswise into ½ inch rounds

3 tomatoes, sliced

5 cloves garlic, minced

3 tablespoons fresh basil leaves, sliced

½ teaspoon dried oregano

Preheat oven to 350 degrees F.

Cover bottom of a baking dish with pasta sauce. Place half of the eggplant slices on the sauce, top with tomato slices and the remaining eggplant slices. Sprinkle garlic, basil and oregano on top.

Cover baking dish with foil and bake for 30 minutes. Uncover and bake for an additional 10 minutes or until eggplant is tender.

CALORIES 160; PROTEIN 6g; CARBOHYDRATES 34g; SUGARS 14g; TOTAL FAT 2g; SATURATED FAT 0.3g; SODIUM 41mg; FIBER 12g

Raw Vegetables with Hummus (from Day 13 lunch)

Fresh or frozen strawberries for dessert

DAY 15

If you eat standard American food, you will inevitably develop standard American diseases.

BREAKFAST

BLUEBERRY NUT STEEL-CUT OATS
1 SERVING

1 cup water

¼ cup steel-cut oats (see note)

½ cup diced apple

1 tablespoon ground flax seeds

½ cup fresh or frozen blueberries

1 tablespoon chopped walnuts or pecans

In a saucepan, bring water to a boil and stir in all ingredients, except blueberries and nuts. Reduce heat, cover, and simmer for 15 minutes or until oats are tender and water is absorbed, stirring occasionally. Stir in blueberries and nuts and heat for another minute.

Note: To make with old-fashioned rolled oats instead of steel cut, use ½ cup oats and reduce cooking time to 5 minutes.

CALORIES 377; PROTEIN 11g; CARBOHYDRATES 52g; SUGARS 14 g; TOTAL FAT 16g; SATURATED FAT 1.2g; SODIUM 13mg; FIBER 11g

LUNCH

FIESTA STUFFER WRAP (or leftover Lentil Quinoa Salad from Day 14)
1 SERVING

1 cup very finely shredded collard greens

2 tablespoons low-sodium salsa

2 tablespoons raw almond butter

2 tablespoons fresh cilantro, minced

½ teaspoon ground cumin

½ teaspoon chili powder

1 (100% whole grain) pita or flour tortilla

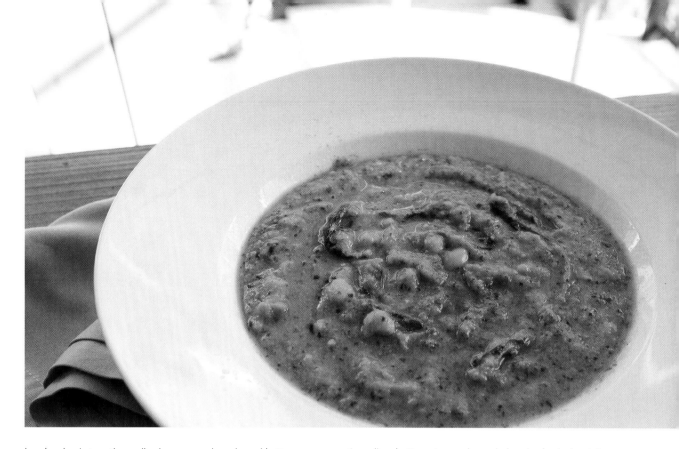

In a bowl, mix together collard greens, salsa, almond butter, cilantro, cumin and chili powder.

Serve stuffed into a whole grain pita or enclosed in a wrap.

CALORIES 305; PROTEIN 11g; CARBOHYDRATES 29g; SUGARS 2g; TOTAL FAT 18g; SATURATED FAT 1.4g; SODIUM 145mg; FIBER 8g

Pineapple or other fruit for dessert

DINNER

BUTTERNUT GINGER SOUP
3 SERVINGS

¾ cup water

1 cup unsweetened soy, hemp or almond milk

2 cups no-salt-added or low-sodium vegetable broth

2 carrots, sliced

3 celery stalks, sliced

1 small onion, sliced

1 teaspoon minced, peeled ginger

1 medium butternut squash, peeled and cubed, about 4 cups (see note)

1 cup sliced mushrooms

1 cup cooked (or low-sodium/no-salt-added canned) white beans, any variety

3 ounces chopped kale or spinach

Place water, non-dairy milk, vegetable broth, carrots, celery, onions, ginger and butternut squash in a large soup pot. Bring to a boil, reduce heat and simmer for 30 minutes or until squash is tender. Transfer to a food processor or blender, and blend until smooth. Return to pot.

Add mushrooms and beans, bring to a simmer and cook for 20 minutes. Add kale or spinach and continue cooking until greens are wilted.

Note: To save time, try precut or frozen butternut squash.

CALORIES 335; PROTEIN 14g; CARBOHYDRATES 72g; SUGARS 13g; TOTAL FAT 2g; SATURATED FAT 0.4g; SODIUM 172mg; FIBER 15g

Men: Have 2 servings of Butternut Ginger Soup.

DAYS 16-20
SHOPPING LIST

This shopping list assumes that all recipes in the meal plan will be made. Menus frequently include fruit for dessert and will mention a specific fruit as an example. That fruit is used for the shopping list.

Check your refrigerator, freezer and pantry before shopping. You may have items leftover from Days 1-15 that you can use. Make sure you also have all the items listed in the Stock Your Pantry list.

FRESH PRODUCE

VEGETABLES

- [ ] 16 ounces mixed salad greens (about 16 cups)
- [ ] 1 head romaine lettuce
- [ ] 9 ounces kale (about 16 cups; increase to 18 cups for men)
- [ ] 10 ounces kale, collards or other greens
- [ ] 3 ounces spinach (about 3 cups)
- [ ] Your choice of a 2 green vegetables to equal 2 cups cooked for each (could also buy frozen)
- [ ] Your choice of a green or non-green vegetable to equal 2 cups cooked (could also buy frozen)
- [ ] 3 medium zucchini
- [ ] 2 green bell peppers
- [ ] 1 red bell pepper
- [ ] Small red cabbage
- [ ] Small eggplant
- [ ] Butternut squash (need 2 cups chopped)
- [ ] Head of cauliflower
- [ ] 5 ounces white or cremini mushrooms
- [ ] 5 medium tomatoes

- [ ] 1 (2 for men) avocado
- [ ] 2 carrots
- [ ] 1 bulb garlic
- [ ] 6 yellow onions
- [ ] 2 red onions
- [ ] Ginger (need ½ inch piece)
- [ ] Chives
- [ ] Parsley
- [ ] Basil

FRUIT

- [ ] 2 ½ cup blueberries (could also buy frozen)
- [ ] 1 cup strawberries (could also buy frozen)
- [ ] 2 ½ cups pineapple chunks (could also buy frozen)
- [ ] 1 (2 for men) apple
- [ ] 1 orange
- [ ] 2 kiwi
- [ ] Small bunch of grapes
- [ ] 4 bananas
- [ ] 1 lemon

REFRIGERATED

- [ ] 6 ½ cups unsweetened, unflavored soy, hemp or almond milk
- [ ] 15 ounces extra firm tofu
- [ ] 4 ounces wild caught salmon or 6 ounces of tempeh
- [ ] Shrimp or chicken (to yield 4 ounces cooked), optional

FROZEN

This list does not include vegetables and fruit listed under fresh produce list that have a frozen option.

- [ ] Corn (need ½ cup)
- [ ] Cherries (need 1 cup) any left from Days 11-15?
- [ ] Mixed berries (need 2 cups)
- [ ] Peaches (need 2 cups)

SHELF STABLE

BEANS

It is assumed that canned, low-sodium or no-salt-added beans will be used. If you opt to start with dry beans, 1 cup of dry beans will yield about 3 cups of cooked beans.

- [ ] 3 (15 ounce) cans chickpeas
- [ ] 2 (15 ounce) cans red pinto or kidney beans
- [ ] 2 (15 ounce) cans any variety white beans
- [ ] 1 (15 ounce) can cannellini or any other bean
- [ ] 1 (15 ounce can black beans
- [ ] Shelled edamame (need 1 cup; could substitute other beans)

OTHER

Choose tomato products packaged in BPA-free materials.

- [ ] 1 (32 ounce) cartons no-salt-added or low-sodium vegetable broth (need about 3 ½ cups)
- [ ] No-salt-added diced tomatoes (need 4 ½ cups)
- [ ] Low-sodium pasta sauce (need 1 ½ cups)
- [ ] Tomato paste (need 1 tablespoon)
- [ ] Almond extract

DAY 16

When you eat a nutrient-rich diet, you are eating more food volume, more food by weight, and more high-water content food. You will feel fuller after a meal even though you are eating fewer calories overall and less high-calorie food.

BREAKFAST

CHICKPEA CEREAL
1 SERVING

¾ cup cooked chickpeas
1 banana, sliced
½ cup blueberries or other berries
1 teaspoon ground chia seeds.
⅓ cup unsweetened soy, hemp or almond milk

Combine ingredients in a cereal bowl.

CALORIES 378; PROTEIN 14g; CARBOHYDRATES 73g; SUGARS 28g; TOTAL FAT 6g; SATURATED FAT 0.6g; SODIUM 73mg; FIBER 15g

Men: Add a ¼ cup of raw nuts.

LUNCH

Big Salad with Ginger Almond Dressing
(Include mixed salad greens, tomatoes, shredded red cabbage and your choice of edamame or other beans)

GINGER ALMOND DRESSING
3 SERVINGS

½ cup raw almonds or ¼ cup raw almond butter
¼ cup unsweetened soy, hemp or almond milk
¼ cup water
2 tablespoons rice vinegar
1 tablespoon unhulled sesame seeds

2 regular dates or 1 Medjool date, pitted
1 clove garlic, chopped
½-inch piece fresh ginger, peeled

Blend all ingredients in a high-powered blender until creamy. Add more water if needed to adjust consistency.

CALORIES 182; PROTEIN 6g; CARBOHYDRATES 10g; SUGARS 6g; TOTAL FAT 14g; SATURATED FAT 1.2g; SODIUM 14mg; FIBER 3.1g

Men: Add sliced avocado to salad.

Orange or other fruit for dessert

DINNER

LEMON CAULIFLOWER RISOTTO
(with optional chicken or shrimp)
2 SERVINGS

½ onion, diced
2 cloves garlic, finely chopped
½ cup low-sodium or no-salt-added vegetable broth
6 cups very finely chopped (riced) cauliflower florets
½ organic lemon, juiced and zested
1 tablespoon nutritional yeast
2 cups spinach, finely sliced
¼ cup raw almond butter
2 tablespoons sliced chives, divided

Water sauté the onion and garlic in 2-3 tablespoons of water, stirring often, until tender, about 5 minutes. Add the vegetable broth and cauliflower and sauté for 3 minutes. Add all other ingredients

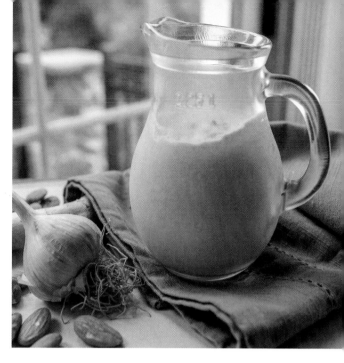

except 1 tablespoon of the chives and cook for 3 more minutes or until cauliflower is al dente. Sprinkle the remaining chives over the risotto.

CALORIES 324; PROTEIN 16g; CARBOHYDRATES 30g; SUGARS 9g; TOTAL FAT 19g; SATURATED FAT 1.6g; SODIUM 160mg; FIBER 12g

Optional: Top with 2 ounces of cooked shrimp or shredded chicken per serving.

Your choice of a cooked green vegetable.

> **Tip:** Steaming is a quick and gentle cooking method that allows valuable nutrients to be retained in the food. It is better than boiling which causes nutrients to be lost in the cooking water. Don't steam vegetables until they are very soft; steam them only until they start to become tender but still retain some firmness.

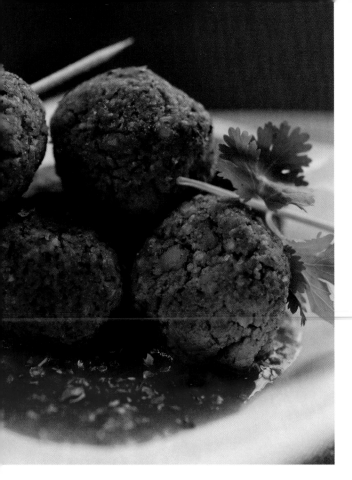

DAY 17

Much of the modern world today suffers from high-calorie malnutrition. This means that although the foods we are eating are rich in calories, they contain insufficient micronutrients.

BREAKFAST

CHOCOLATE ALMOND SMOOTHIE
1 SERVING

2 cups chopped kale
½ cup unsweetened soy, hemp or almond milk
¼ cup water
½ banana
1 cup frozen cherries
2 tablespoons raw almonds
2 tablespoons natural cocoa powder
1 tablespoon ground flax seeds
1 teaspoon almond extract

Blend ingredients in a high-powered blender until smooth and creamy.

CALORIES 368; PROTEIN 17g; CARBOHYDRATES 57g; SUGARS 22; TOTAL FAT 17g; SATURATED FAT 2g; SODIUM 81mg; FIBER 14g

Men: Use the whole banana.

LUNCH

QUICK AND EASY BEAN SALAD
(or leftover Lemon Cauliflower Risotto from Day 16 dinner served on a bed of mixed greens)
1 SERVING

1 cup cooked cannellini or other beans
¼ cup chopped red onion
1 tomato, chopped
2 tablespoons chopped parsley
1 tablespoon balsamic vinegar
½ teaspoon no-salt seasoning blend such as Dr. Fuhrman's VegiZest or Mrs. Dash
5 cups mixed salad greens

Mix all ingredients except salad greens in a bowl. Serve bean mixture on top of the greens.

CALORIES 364; PROTEIN 25g; CARBOHYDRATES 67g; SUGARS 9g; TOTAL FAT 1.9g; SATURATED FAT 0.4g; SODIUM 131mg; FIBER 19.8g

Men: Add ¼ cup raw nuts or seeds.

2 kiwi or other fruit for dessert

DINNER

TOFU MEATBALLS
2 SERVINGS

8 ounces extra firm tofu, drained
¼ cup ground walnuts
¼ cup old-fashioned oats, blended to make coarse crumbs
2 tablespoons whole wheat flour (or more old-fashioned oats)
¼ cup minced onion
½ teaspoon dried oregano, or to taste
½ teaspoon dried basil, or to taste
1 teaspoon Bragg Liquid Aminos or low-sodium soy sauce
1 ½ cups low-sodium pasta sauce

Mix all ingredients very well, using hands if necessary.

Form into 2-inch balls. Place on a baking pan that has been lightly oiled or lined with parchment paper. Bake at 350 degrees F for 30-35 minutes or until golden.

Serve topped with low-sodium pasta sauce.

CALORIES 211; PROTEIN 12g; CARBOHYDRATES 19g; SUGARS 2.7g; TOTAL FAT 10.6g; SATURATED FAT 1.2g; SODIUM 156mg; FIBER 3.5g

Onion and Garlic-Braised Greens (recipe from Day 5 dinner)

BERRY BLEND SHERBET
3 SERVINGS

1 cup unsweetened soy, hemp or almond milk
1 frozen banana (see note)
2 cups frozen mixed berries
2 cups frozen peach slices

Blend ingredients in a high-powered blender until smooth. Portion leftover servings individually and store in freezer.

Note: Freeze ripe bananas at least 8 hours in advance. Peel bananas and seal in a plastic bag before freezing.

CALORIES 146; PROTEIN 4g; CARBOHYDRATES 31g; SUGARS 20; TOTAL FAT 2g; SATURATED FAT 0.3g; SODIUM 32mg; FIBER 5.4g

You can have the leftover sherbet as a lunch or dinner dessert on Days 18 or 19. Allow it to soften at room temperature for a few minutes.

DAY 18

Type 2 diabetes almost never occurs in people who eat healthfully, exercise regularly and have a low percentage of body fat. The disease hardly existed in prior centuries when food was less abundant or when high-calorie, low-nutrient food was not available.

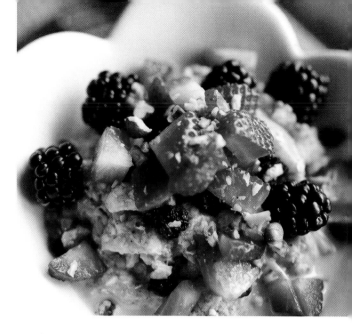

BREAKFAST

BUCKWHEAT AND BERRIES CEREAL
1 SERVING

¼ cup raw buckwheat groats, rinsed (see note)
½ cup unsweetened soy, hemp or almond milk
¼ teaspoon cinnamon
¼ teaspoon alcohol-free vanilla extract
1 apple, chopped or grated
½ tablespoon raw almond or cashew butter
1 tablespoon chia seeds
½ cup fresh or thawed frozen blueberries or other berries

Place buckwheat, non-dairy milk, cinnamon and vanilla in a pot. Bring to a boil, reduce heat, cover and simmer for 6 minutes or until groats are soft but not mushy and almost all liquid is absorbed. Stir in apple, nut butter and chia seeds and simmer for another minute.

Stir in berries. Add additional non-dairy milk if desired. May be refrigerated and eaten cold or reheated.

Note: Buckwheat groats are seeds from the buckwheat plant. They are unrelated to wheat and do not contain gluten. Choose raw buckwheat groats, not kasha, which is toasted.

CALORIES 369; PROTEIN 10g; CARBOHYDRATES 65g; SUGARS 21g; TOTAL FAT 10g; SATURATED FAT 1.0g; SODIUM 101mg; FIBER 12g

LUNCH

CREAMY ZOODLES
2 SERVINGS

3 medium zucchini

1 ripe avocado, peeled and pitted
½ cup fresh basil leaves
1 tablespoon lemon juice
1 clove garlic
⅛ teaspoon ground black pepper
1 teaspoon Bragg Liquid Aminos
1 tablespoon water
1 tablespoon lemon zest

Use a julienne peeler (or a spiral slicer or a regular vegetable peeler) to make long, thin strips of zucchini that resemble spaghetti.

To make the sauce, combine avocado, basil, lemon juice, garlic, black pepper, Bragg Liquid Aminos and water in a food processor or high-powered blender and process until smooth and creamy. Add additional water if needed to adjust consistency.

Toss the uncooked (or lightly steamed) zucchini noodles with the sauce. Top with lemon zest.

CALORIES 172; PROTEIN 6g; CARBOHYDRATES 17g; SUGARS 7.9g; TOTAL FAT 11.5g; SATURATED FAT 1.7g; SODIUM 85mg; FIBER 8.1g;

Men: Add raw vegetables with low-sodium salsa

Grapes or other fruit

DINNER

TWO BEAN CHILI (any frozen leftovers from Day 10?)
4 SERVINGS

1 cup chopped onion
½ cup chopped green bell pepper
1 clove garlic, chopped
¾ cup water

2 tablespoons tomato paste
1 tablespoon chili powder
2 teaspoons ground cumin
¼ teaspoon black pepper
1 ½ cups cooked black beans or 1 (15 ounce) can low-sodium or no-salt-added black beans, drained
3 cups cooked red pinto or kidney beans or 2 (15 ounce) cans low-sodium or no-salt-added red beans, drained
2 cups low-sodium or no-salt-added vegetable broth
1 ½ cups diced tomatoes
½ cup frozen corn kernels
1 tablespoon yellow cornmeal

Water sauté onion and bell pepper in a soup pot until almost tender. Add garlic and cook for another minute. Stir in water, tomato paste, chili powder, cumin, black pepper, beans, vegetable broth, diced tomatoes and corn and bring to a boil. Reduce heat, cover and simmer for 10 minutes. Stir in cornmeal and cook for an additional two minutes.

CALORIES 338; PROTEIN 20g; CARBOHYDRATES 64g; SUGARS 6g; TOTAL FAT 2g; SATURATED FAT 0.3g; SODIUM 120mg; FIBER 19g

Men: Have 2 servings of Two Bean Chili.

Your choice of a cooked green or other high-nutrient vegetable. (The high-nutrient, non-green vegetables are: tomatoes, onions, mushrooms, cauliflower, eggplant and red peppers.)

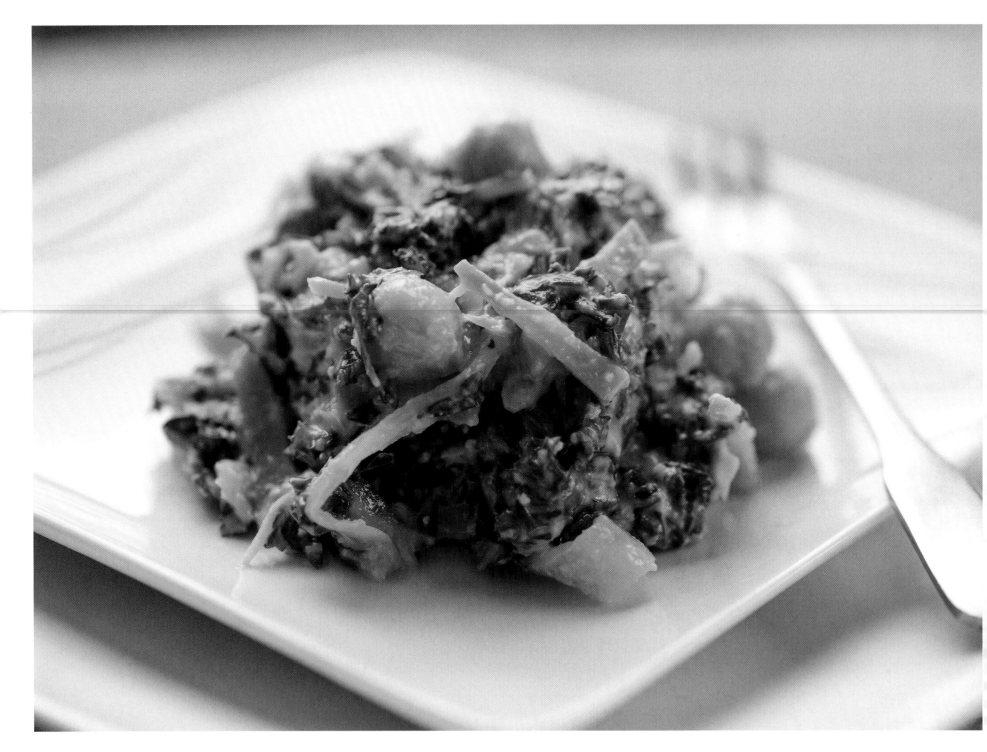

DAY 19

Instead of teaching how excellent nutrition can prevent disease, typical diabetes care is focused on the wrong thing—monitoring blood sugar to determine when it is necessary to adjust medications.

BREAKFAST

TOFU SCRAMBLE WITH TOMATOES AND PEPPERS
1 SERVING

½ cup chopped green or red pepper

¼ cup chopped onion

1 clove garlic, chopped

1 cup diced tomatoes

7 ounces extra-firm tofu, drained and crumbled

1 cup firmly-packed spinach

½ teaspoon garlic powder

¼ teaspoon turmeric

¼ teaspoon red pepper flakes or ⅛ teaspoon chipotle powder, if desired

Heat 2-3 tablespoons water in a large skillet and water sauté peppers, onion and garlic until tender. Add remaining ingredients and cook for another five minutes.

CALORIES 258; PROTEIN 22g; CARBOHYDRATES 23g; SUGARS 9g; TOTAL FAT 10g; SATURATED FAT 1.3g; SODIUM 90mg; FIBER 7g

Men: Add a Waldorf Blended Salad (Day 14 breakfast)

LUNCH

CALIFORNIA CREAMED KALE AND CHICKPEAS
4 SERVINGS

½ cup raw cashews

1 cup unsweetened soy, almond or hemp milk

1 clove garlic

1 large onion, thinly sliced

2 carrots, finely chopped

1 ½ cups cooked chickpeas or 1 (15 ounce) can no-salt-added or low-sodium chickpeas, drained

1 bunch (about 1 pound) kale, tough stems removed, leaves thinly sliced

¼ teaspoon crushed red pepper or to taste

Place cashews, non-dairy milk and garlic in a high-powered blender and blend until smooth. Set aside.

Heat 2-3 tablespoons water in a large skillet and water sauté the onion and carrots for 5 minutes, or until softened. Stir in the chickpeas. Gradually add the kale and sauté until kale starts to wilt, adding additional water as needed to prevent sticking. Cover and cook until kale is tender, about 10 minutes.

Stir in cashew sauce and crushed red pepper. Cook, uncovered for 2-3 minutes until heated through.

CALORIES 335; PROTEIN 16g; CARBOHYDRATES 45g; SUGARS 9g; TOTAL FAT 11g; SATURATED FAT 1.8g; SODIUM 70mg; FIBER 11g

Blueberries or other fruit for dessert

DINNER

ROASTED VEGETABLE SALAD TOPPED WITH SALMON (or Baked Tempeh Strips)
2 SERVINGS

1 red pepper, cut into ½ inch pieces

1 small eggplant, cut into ½ inch pieces

2 cups butternut squash, peeled and cut into ½ inch pieces

2 tablespoons balsamic vinegar

1 tablespoon low-sodium vegetable broth

2 cloves garlic, minced

1 teaspoon Bragg Liquid Aminos or low-sodium soy sauce

black pepper, to taste

4 ounces wild-caught salmon (see note for tempeh option)

⅛ teaspoon garlic powder

6 cups mixed salad greens

Preheat oven to 400 degrees F. Lightly coat a large baking pan using a paper towel moistened with olive oil. Place vegetables in pan. In a small bowl, combine broth, vinegar, garlic, Bragg Liquid Aminos, and black pepper and toss with vegetables. Roast in oven for 18 - 20 minutes, until tender, stirring occasionally.

Cut salmon into 2 pieces. Season with garlic powder and black pepper. Place salmon, skin side down on a non-stick baking sheet. Bake at 400 degrees F until salmon is cooked through, about 12-15 minutes.

Place mixed greens on serving plates. Top with roasted vegetables and salmon.

Note: Baked Tempeh Strips may be substituted for the salmon.

To prepare Baked Tempeh Strips: Cut 6 ounces of tempeh into very thin 1-inch strips. Whisk together 3 tablespoons wine vinegar, ½ cup water, 2 tablespoons natural, unsalted peanut butter and 1 teaspoon chopped fresh ginger or garlic. Place sliced tempeh in a baking dish, add the peanut mixture and marinate for 30 minutes. Bake at 300 degrees F for 20 minutes or until marinade is absorbed.

CALORIES 223; PROTEIN 19g; CARBOHYDRATES 31g; SUGARS 10g; TOTAL FAT 4g; SATURATED FAT 1.0g; SODIUM 186mg; FIBER 10g

Grapes or other fruit for dessert

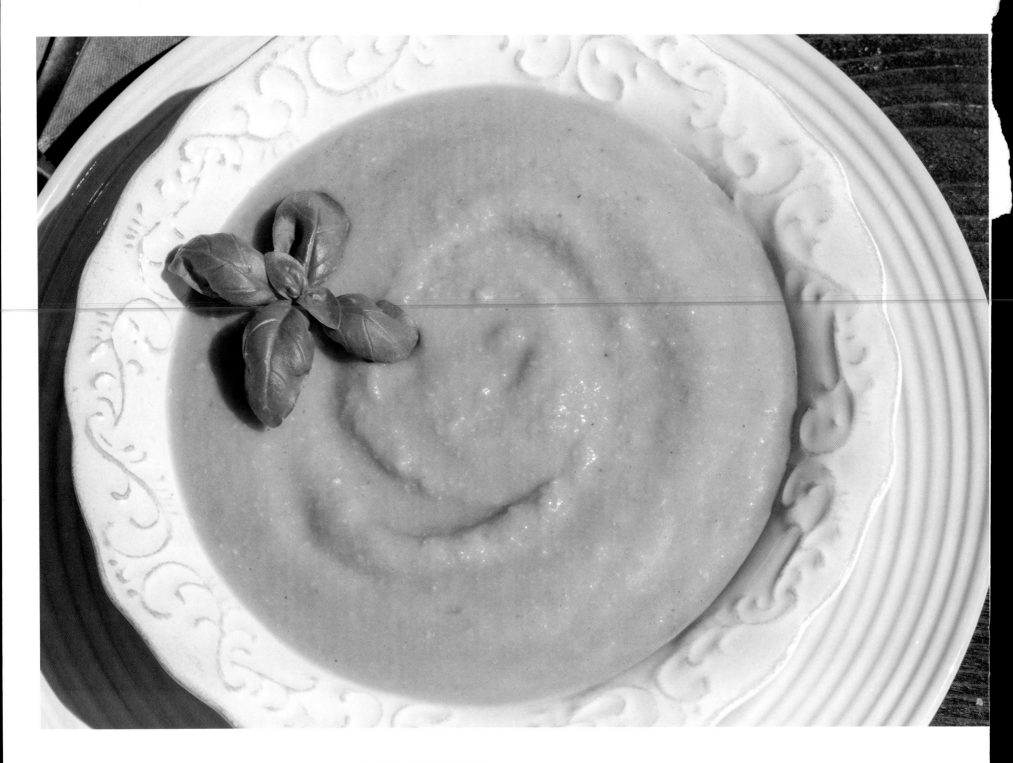

DAY 20

Food can either kill or heal — the choice is yours.

BREAKFAST

NO-COOK STRAWBERRY OATMEAL
1 SERVING

⅓ cup old-fashioned rolled oats

1 tablespoon chia seeds

⅔ cup unsweetened soy, hemp or almond milk

1 cup fresh or thawed frozen strawberries, sliced (or blueberries, cherries or sliced peaches)

2 tablespoons chopped walnuts

Combine the oats, chia seeds and non-dairy milk. Soak for at least 30 minutes or overnight. Stir in sliced strawberries and walnuts.

CALORIES 334; PROTEIN 13g; CARBOHYDRATES 39g; SUGARS 9g; TOTAL FAT 16g; SATURATED FAT 1.8g; SODIUM 64mg; FIBER 11g

LUNCH

Big Salad with Easy Balsamic Almond Dressing, topped with Chickpea Popcorn (Include romaine lettuce, tomatoes, red onions and lightly sautéed mushrooms)

EASY BALSAMIC ALMOND DRESSING
1 SERVING

2 tablespoons water

1 tablespoon plus 1 teaspoon balsamic vinegar

1 tablespoon raw almond butter

¼ teaspoon onion powder

¼ teaspoon garlic powder

⅛ teaspoon dried oregano

⅛ teaspoon dried basil

Whisk water, vinegar and almond butter together until mixture is smooth and almond butter is evenly dispersed. Mix in remaining ingredients.

CALORIES 127; PROTEIN 4g; CARBOHYDRATES 9g; SUGARS 5g; TOTAL FAT 9g; SATURATED FAT 0.7g; SODIUM 10mg; FIBER 2g

Men: Add a leftover soup or bean burger.

ITALIAN CHICKPEA POPCORN
6 SERVINGS

1 ½ cups cooked chickpeas or 1 (15 ounce) can no-salt-added or low-sodium chickpeas, drained

1 teaspoon ground cumin

1 teaspoon garlic powder

1 teaspoon oregano

pinch cayenne pepper, or to taste

Preheat oven to 350 degrees F. Mix chickpeas with remaining ingredients. Spread on a parchment paper lined baking sheet and bake for 40 - 45 minutes or until crispy, stirring occasionally.

CALORIES 71; PROTEIN 4g; CARBOHYDRATES 12g; SUGARS 2g; TOTAL FAT 1g; SATURATED FAT 0.1g; SODIUM 4mg; FIBER 3g

DINNER

CREAM OF TOMATO SOUP
4 SERVINGS

1 onion, chopped

1 green pepper, chopped

½ cup no-salt-added or low-sodium vegetable broth

3 cups (about 26 ounces) diced tomatoes and juice

3 cups cooked white beans, any variety or 2 (15 ounce) cans low-sodium or no-salt-added beans

¼ cup balsamic vinegar

½ cup raw cashews or ¼ cup raw cashew butter

1 cup unsweetened soy, hemp or almond milk

Combine vegetable broth with onion and green pepper in a large sauté pan. Bring to a boil, reduce heat and simmer until vegetables are tender and broth is almost boiled off. Add diced tomatoes with juice, beans and vinegar. Bring to a boil, reduce heat, cover and simmer for 45 minutes.

Transfer to a high-powered blender, add cashews and non-dairy milk and blend until smooth. Return to pot to reheat.

CALORIES 347; PROTEIN 16g; CARBOHYDRATES 54g; SUGARS 10g; TOTAL FAT 9g; SATURATED FAT 1.5g; SODIUM 16mg; FIBER 18g

Your choice of a steamed or water-sautéed green vegetable (add your green vegetable to the soup if you prefer)

BANANA PINEAPPLE PUDDING
2 SERVINGS

1 ripe banana

1 cup fresh or frozen pineapple chunks

Blend ingredients together until smooth.

CALORIES 93; PROTEIN 1g; CARBOHYDRATES 24g; SUGARS 15g; TOTAL FAT 0.2g; SATURATED FAT 0g; SODIUM 1mg; FIBER 3g

CONGRATULATIONS!

YOU HAVE COMPLETED DAY 20!

Congratulations on completing Day 20 of the *Transformation 20 Diabetes Program*! By now, if you have faithfully adhered to the program, you have undoubtedly made great progress in lowering your glucose levels, reducing your medication, regaining your energy level and restoring your health. All in just a few, short weeks. Good for you — you are on your way! I hope you are encouraged by the improvements you have made to your health. Don't stop now. Use your results as momentum to push yourself forward to accomplish even more.

You can, and should, make these changes permanent. You may want to repeat the menus for one or more additional 20-day cycles. You could also log onto *DrFuhrman.com* to try our other exciting recipes or you can begin to design your own menus based on my Nutritarian principles. And, don't worry. Help is always available in navigating the road to better health: You can learn more about the Nutritarian eating style by reading one or more of my books or by becoming a member of my website, *DrFuhrman.com*. Either option will give you helpful tips, cooking advice and additional compelling reasons why eating this way is so important to prevent chronic illness, maintain superior health and increase longevity.

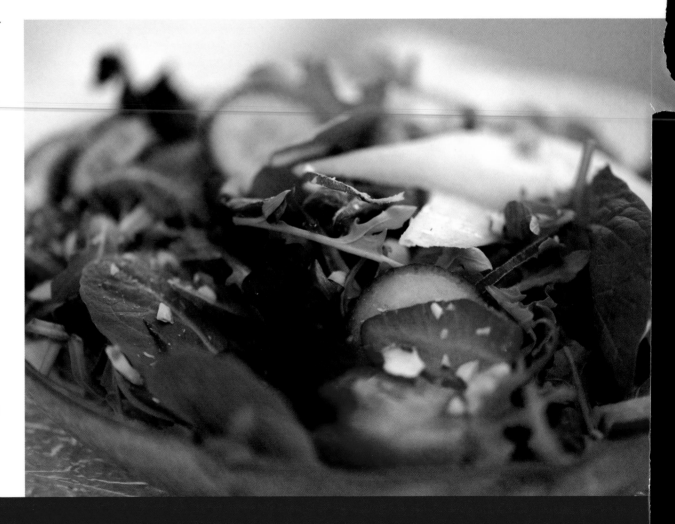